COMMUNITY LIBRARY

3 2301 00193012 6

"*Yoga and Fertility* is a great resource for women seeking to optimize their fertility. Yoga provides an important adjunct to the mind/body approach to fertility proven beneficial to reduce stress and improve mental and physical well-being. By presenting the 'how' and the 'why' of each exercise, the authors provide the reader with the knowledge, insight and encourage
of this powerful tool."

R
Sea

Seattle, WA

"A wonderfully rich and concise manual. Lynn Jensen and Jill Petigara provide an easy to follow program to take you through poses that enhance each phase of the menstrual cycle, regardless of your familiarity with yoga. Beginner, intermediate, or advanced, you will find detailed photos, descriptions, and reasons for these healing exercises."

Randine Lewis, L.Ac., Ph.D.
FABORM
www.thefertilesoul.com

"Only those who dare to plunge to their depths can re-emerge triumphant, wise and fulfilled. Lynn Jensen and Jill Petigara both longed to be mothers. Their struggle with infertility and the failure of medical intervention turned them back on themselves and to their Yoga practice. Finally, letting go of all expectations, a perfect baby arrived for each of them. The gratitude they both found in the gift of their babies led them to assist other women struggling with infertility. This is a beautiful and informative book that will give hope and help to many women."

Angela Farmer, International Yoga Teacher

"Those who are interested in practicing yoga in the context of their path to parenthood, whether they are yoga novices or long-time practitioners, will find in this book a very easy-to-follow guide to poses, breathing, and relaxation. The photographs and descriptions of poses and sequences are excellent. Also, by including a rationale for each pose, the authors engage the reader in an active understanding of the function of each pose and how it may be helpful during each part of a woman's cycle. These aspects of the book are excellent, but perhaps the most important quality of the book is that it focuses on the mind-body connection and encourages those seeking fertility support to begin a journey of greater understanding, compassion, and healing for the self. Miracles are not promised, but 'success' is viewed as progress along the path of increasing wellness and acceptance, no matter the outcome."

Cathryn Booth-LaForce, Ph.D., RYT
Professor, University of Washington

"With their extensive training in yoga and personal struggles with starting their families, Jill Petigara and Lynn Jensen have created an informative guide for people who are trying to conceive and wish to incorporate yoga into their own journey to parenthood."

Lora Shahine, M.D., F.A.C.O.G.
Pacific NW Fertility and IVF Specialists

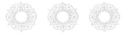

"*Yoga and Fertility* is a terrific resource for women who are trying to overcome fertility challenges or just starting to prepare for conception. I specialize in medical nutrition therapy for reproductive nutrition and my patients want to know they are doing everything possible to conceive a healthy child. The fertility journey can be stressful and often overwhelming and I frequently recommend yoga. What a great resource for women to learn more about the benefits of fertility yoga, with detailed instructions, great illustrations and explanations!"

Judy Simon MS,RD Mind Body Nutrition, PLLC
And University Washington Medical Center Faculty and Dietitian
www.mind-body-nutrition.com

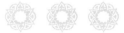

"*Yoga and Fertility* shows us how to apply ancient and time tested methods that can truly heal, rejuvenate and strengthen our body, mind and spirit. Its straightforward and holistic approach shares key teachings on how to establish our body's innate capacities. More than a tool to help women achieve their dream of getting pregnant, having a healthy pregnancy, and finally bringing a child into the world, *Yoga and Fertility* provides guidance that can benefit men or women, in other words, anyone wanting to have more of the life they truly desire."

Rod Stryker, Founder of ParaYoga, author of *The Four Desires*

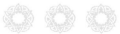

"Focusing the mind and body through a regular yoga practice reduces stress and improves health. This is a great benefit for women undergoing demanding fertility treatments. I've been fortunate to have Lynn's *Yoga and Fertility* class available for my patients locally and am so glad that Lynn and Jill have decided to share their expertise with a wider audience. I know this book will be a valuable resource and recommend it highly."

Angela Thyer, M.D.
Seattle Reproductive Medicine

"An amazing step-by-step guide to the most beneficial yoga postures for fertility, scientifically shown to elicit the relaxation response. Lynn Jensen and Jill Petigara's *Yoga and Fertility* is a key ingredient to nourishing reproductive health on a cellular level."

Kathryn Simmons Flynn, Founder of Fertile Foods and author of *Cooking for Fertility*
www.fertilefoods.com

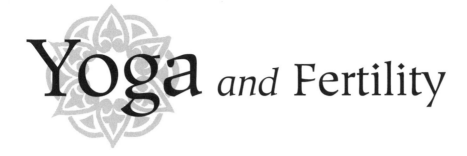

Yoga *and* Fertility

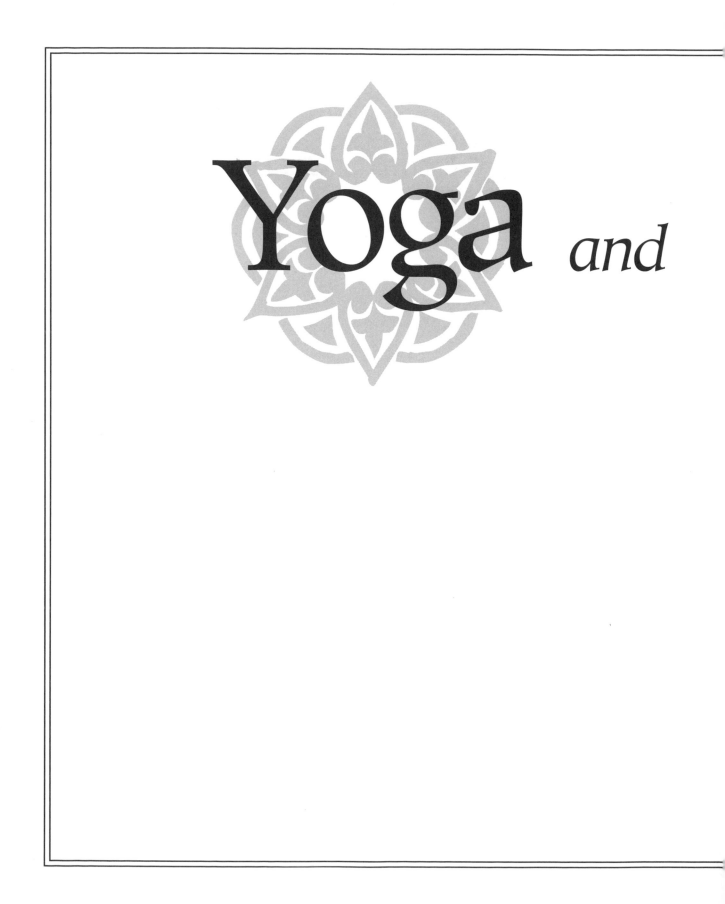

Yoga *and*

Fertility

A Journey to Health and Healing

JILL MAHRLIG PETIGARA, E-RYT, MA

AND

LYNN JENSEN, E-RYT, RPYT, MBA

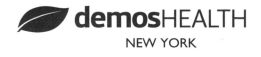
demosHEALTH

NEW YORK

Visit our website at www.demoshealth.com

ISBN: 978-1-936303-32-8
e-book ISBN: 9781617051111

Acquisitions Editor: Noreen Henson
Compositor: diacriTech

© 2013 by Jill Mahrlig Petigara and Lynn Jensen. All rights reserved. This book is protected by copyright. No part of it may be reproduced, stored in a retrieval system, or transmitted in any form or by any means, electronic, mechanical, photocopying, recording, or otherwise, without the prior written permission of the publisher.

Medical information provided by Demos Health, in the absence of a visit with a health care professional, must be considered as an educational service only. This book is not designed to replace a physician's independent judgment about the appropriateness or risks of a procedure or therapy for a given patient. Our purpose is to provide you with information that will help you make your own health care decisions.

The information and opinions provided here are believed to be accurate and sound, based on the best judgment available to the authors, editors, and publisher, but readers who fail to consult appropriate health authorities assume the risk of injuries. The publisher is not responsible for errors or omissions. The editors and publisher welcome any reader to report to the publisher any discrepancies or inaccuracies noticed.

Library of Congress Cataloging-in-Publication Data.

Petigara, Jill Mahrlig.
  Yoga and fertility : a journey to health and healing / Jill Mahrlig Petigara and Lynn Jensen.
    p. cm.
  ISBN 978-1-936303-32-8
  1. Hatha yoga. 2. Fertility, Human. 3. Women—Health and hygiene. 4. Self-care, Health. I. Jensen, Lynn. II. Title.
  RA781.7.P478 2012
  613.7'046—dc23

                                                                                    2012030128

Special discounts on bulk quantities of Demos Health books are available to corporations, professional associations, pharmaceutical companies, health care organizations, and other qualifying groups. For details, please contact:

Special Sales Department
Demos Medical Publishing, LLC
11 West 42nd Street, 15th Floor
New York, NY 10036
Phone: 800-532-8663 or 212-683-0072
Fax: 212-941-7842
E-mail: rsantana@demosmedpub.com

Printed in the United States of America by Bang Printing
12 13 14 15 / 5 4 3 2 1

Jill and Lynn would like to dedicate this book to all of our students, past, present and future, and to anyone who has ever faced fertility challenges.

Contents

Foreword   Carol Knoph, MEd, LMHC   xv

Acknowledgments   xvii

Introduction: Why We Wrote This Book   xix

CHAPTER 1. WHAT IS YOGA FOR FERTILITY?   1

General Yoga Benefits   3

Yoga for Fertility Benefits   3

CHAPTER 2. WHO CAN BENEFIT FROM YOGA FOR FERTILITY?   13

Just Starting Out   13

Unexplained Infertility   13

PCOS   14

Endometriosis   14

Miscarriage   15

Is Yoga for Fertility Helpful for Men?   16

The Research: Is Yoga for Fertility Effective?   17

CHAPTER 3. GETTING STARTED WITH YOGA FOR FERTILITY   19

Getting Started   20

Deciding Where to Begin in This Book   21

How Much Time and How Often Should You Do These Routines?   22

Keeping a Journal   22

Basic Yoga Principles   23

CHAPTER 4. ROUTINES FOR THE FIRST HALF OF YOUR CYCLE   27

First Half Basic Routine   28

Summary Flow of First Half Basic Routine   28

POSE DESCRIPTIONS FOR FIRST HALF BASIC ROUTINE   38

    Poses Lying on Your Back   39

    Poses on Hands and Knees   45

    Supine Poses and Lunge Pose   51

    Standing Poses   56

    Seated Poses   62

    Relaxation Poses   67

First Half Intermediate Routine   70

Summary Flow of First Half Intermediate Routine   70

POSE DESCRIPTIONS FOR FIRST HALF INTERMEDIATE ROUTINE   80

    Poses Lying on Your Back   81

    Poses on Hands and Knees   83

    Standing Poses   92

    Supine Poses   100

    More Poses Lying on Your Back   104

    Relaxation Poses   111

CHAPTER 5. ROUTINES FOR THE SECOND HALF OF YOUR CYCLE   115

Second Half Basic Routine   115

Summary Flow of Second Half Basic Routine   116

POSE DESCRIPTIONS FOR SECOND HALF BASIC ROUTINE   126

    Poses Lying on Your Back   127

    Poses on Hands and Knees   136

    Standing Poses   143

    Seated Poses   148

    Relaxation Poses   151

Second Half Intermediate Routine   154

Summary Flow for Second Half Intermediate Routine   154

POSE DESCRIPTIONS FOR SECOND HALF INTERMEDIATE ROUTINE   162

    Poses Lying on Your Back   163

    Poses on Hands and Knees   166

    Standing Poses   171

    Seated Poses   180

    Pre-Relaxation Poses on the Back   184

    Relaxation Poses   187

CHAPTER 6. YOGA ROUTINES FOR ADDITIONAL SITUATIONS   191

Yoga During Your Period   191

Yoga Routine for Your Period   192

    Poses Lying on Your Back   193

    Poses on Hands and Knees   196

    Seated Poses   199

    Relaxation Poses   203

Yoga for Early Pregnancy   204

Cycles Using Assisted Reproductive Technology (ART)   206

YOGA ROUTINE FOR ART CYCLES OR STRESS RELIEF   208

    Poses Lying on Your Back   209

Poses on Hands and Knees   210

Seated Poses   213

More Poses Lying on Your Back   215

Relaxation Poses   219

Adapting Your Yoga Practice in a Class   222

Yoga with Your Partner   223

CHAPTER 7. MORE YOGA PRACTICES FOR FERTILITY SUPPORT   225

Conscious Breathing Practice (Pranayama) for Fertility Support   226

Yoga for Fertility Breathing Practices   228

Meditations and Visualizations for Fertility Support   231

Seated Meditation to Clear the Mind   233

Seated Meditation for Calming   234

Mindful Walking Meditation   235

Passage Meditation   236

Heart-to-Uterus Visualization   237

Affirmations for Fertility Support   238

Vision Boards and Fertility "Altars"   239

Chanting   240

CHAPTER 8. LIFESTYLE CHANGES TO SUPPORT FERTILITY   243

Fertility Nutrition   243

Different Approaches to Fertility Nutrition   244

The Traditional Chinese Medicine Approach   244

The Western Dietician Approach   244

The Food Sensitivities Approach   244

The Ayurvedic Approach   245

The Whole Foods Approach   245

Mindful Eating   247

Nutritional Deficiencies   247

Weight and Fertility   249

Exercise   250

Work and Relationships   253

Top Five Lifestyle Changes for Fertility   253

**CHAPTER 9. USING YOGA WITH OTHER MODALITIES FOR
FERTILITY SUPPORT   255**

Acupuncture   256

Fertility Abdominal Massage   257

Hypnotherapy   258

Counseling and Life Coaching   258

Assisted Reproductive Technology (ART)   258

Suggestions for Friends and Family   260

CHAPTER 10. SUCCESS STORIES   265

Wendy's Story   265

Anna's Story   267

Georgia's Story   269

Suzette's Story   271

Priti's Story   272

Vicky's Story   273

Kathy's Story   274

Nancy's Story   276

Final Thoughts from Jill and Lynn   277

Notes   279

Resources   281

Index   283

Foreword

Yoga and Fertility is an invaluable resource for people trying to conceive; either just beginning to prepare themselves for pregnancy, or for those who have already been trying for some time. Since 2004, I've taught the nationally-recognized mind/body program for fertility developed by Alice D. Domar, Ph.D., at Seattle-area fertility clinics. This innovative program focuses on couples who have not been able to conceive or have a history of miscarriage, and features mind/body techniques such as the relaxation response, cognitive restructuring (i.e., dealing with negative thoughts), lifestyle changes, effective communication and self-nurturance.

One of the highlights during this ten-week program is the Yoga for Fertility session taught by Lynn Jensen. Lynn has brought to my students new ways to help them weather the storm of fertility challenges as well as a way to live life to its fullest during this hopeful time.

The practice of yoga is well known as an antidote for stress. Stress is known to have a negative impact on fertility, so learning the relaxation response is very important for women trying to conceive. When teaching the relaxation response, I find that some women have a difficult time calming their bodies and minds in sitting meditation; their thoughts race and their bodies won't stay still. Yoga is an ideal solution for this problem. Focusing your mind on your body while doing yoga helps to keep you in the present rather than ruminating about the past or worrying about the future. What's more, it also helps relieve muscle tension that builds up from stress.

During fertility treatment, women often feel little control over their lives and bodies. Doctors tell them when to have sex or literally take over their reproductive cycles with medication and procedures. *Yoga and Fertility* can help women get in touch with their bodies in a positive way using gentle poses that coincide with their cycles. You'll find in the book that Lynn and Jill have chosen poses, breathing exercises, and meditations geared toward stimulating or supporting the reproductive system and relieving stress. While waiting for that next cycle to begin or during the very stressful two-week wait for the results of your pregnancy test, yoga is fertility treatment you administer yourself.

Research on exercise and fertility supports mild, low impact exercise, such as yoga for fertility or walking, as an effective type of exercise for women who are trying to get pregnant. I recommend yoga and walking to my students as an alternative to more rigorous exercise during this time.

I think you'll find this book—the only one of its kind to date—to be an important tool to use on your path to parenthood. The extensive knowledge and experience in the field of fertility that Lynn and Jill have is evident in the pages of *Yoga and Fertility*.

What an exciting path you are on, trying to become a parent! I hope that your dreams of building a family are realized soon. *Yoga and Fertility* will offer you a way to do something positive for your mind and body while on your journey to parenthood.

Carol Knoph, MEd, LMHC
Mind/Body Program for Fertility
Peak Health
Seattle, WA

Acknowledgments

Lynn and Jill Would Like to Thank . . .

- All the women who shared their fertility stories, for our chapter on success stories: Anna, Georgia, Priti, Suzette, Wendy, Kathy, Nancy and Vicky (not their real names, but they know who they are!).
- Ricole for sharing her affirmations and ideas on vision boards.
- Every one of our Yoga for Fertility students, who over the years have taught and re-taught the importance of persistence, faith, and supporting one another in our life challenges.
- Janet Michel, RN, LAc, for her vast knowledge of fertility practices, both Eastern and Western, and her contributions to the acupuncture section.

- Sarah Furtek Lawrence, LMP and doula, for information on the Arvigo Techniques of Maya Abdominal Therapy™.
- Nicole Webel Pelly, MD, for providing the information for the section on MTHFR.
- Eliza Truitt, of Eliza Truitt Photography, for her expertise, skill, patience and good humor throughout the photo shoots.
- Daniel Maguire for the generous use of his beautiful yoga studio, SouthEnd Yoga, in Columbia City, Seattle, as the site of our photo shoots.
- Carol Knoph, for her support of yoga for fertility, and for offering to write the Foreword.
- Everyone else who contributed ideas and suggestions for the book—they were much appreciated!

ACKNOWLEDGMENTS

Additional Thanks from Lynn to . . .

- Jill Petigara for offering me the opportunity to work with her, and to finally write the book that has been in my heart (and my bottom drawer) waiting to come out.
- Conner, for being the right child at the right time, and being a constant teacher.
- Bob Smith of the Hatha Yoga Center for sharing his deep knowledge and passion for yoga over many, many years.
- Angela Farmer for opening my eyes to the concept of yoga especially for women.
- Rod Stryker for his brilliant teaching, and his dedication to bringing the ancient wisdom and practices of yoga to Western yogis.
- The many other teachers who have shared their wisdom with me along the way.
- All my family and friends who have been patient with me during the writing process—your support has been invaluable!

Additional Thanks from Jill to . . .

- Lynn Jensen for agreeing to write this book with me after one phone conversation. I could never have done this without you.
- Noreen Henson for asking me to put my program in book form and answering all of our questions along the way.
- My husband Dilip for your unconditional love and support. You are my rock.
- My son Raj who brings more joy to my life than I could have ever imagined possible.
- My parents for all your support and encouragement and being the best grandparents ever.
- Tracey, Doreen, Erica, and Beth Ann—your support has meant the world to me.
- Priya Muthu for asking me to teach Fertility Yoga.
- Dr. Ruijuan Liu for being more than a talented acupuncturist but also a dear friend.
- Jack, Debra, and Dianne at Stillpoint Yoga Studio for giving me a home to teach Fertility Yoga.
- All of my yoga teachers for sharing your wisdom and generosity of heart.

Introduction: Why We Wrote This Book

JILL'S STORY

I have always loved children and found out very early on that I had an ability to relate to them quite effortlessly. Because of this, I became an elementary school teacher and have worked with children of all different age levels for more than half of my life.

As my career evolved to working more with teachers as a consultant and trainer, my stress level increased considerably. I found that yoga was an antidote to all of the stress I was experiencing in my life, both personally and professionally. I not only started practicing yoga regularly, but got certified as a yoga teacher about three years after trying it for the first time.

I was approaching my mid-thirties and accepted the fact that I may never marry or have children when I met my husband, Dilip, on e-Harmony. To be honest, I was only on e-Harmony to pacify my mother who had heard about it on a daytime talk show. Once Dilip and I spoke on the phone, I knew he would become my husband, and we got married just after my 35th birthday.

We threw away the birth control immediately and started trying to conceive a baby. We both had busy schedules at the time but tried to at least be together during ovulation so that we could get moving on this baby business. After a year of trying with no luck, I went to my OB/GYN who recommended I visit a reproductive endocrinologist. I'll never forget that first visit when the doctor told me we were a pretty boring case with just a mild form of PCOS. He was certain that we would get pregnant with some Clomid and an IUI.

I responded well to the medication and everything looked good, but I was not able to get pregnant after three tries of Clomid/IUI. With each failed procedure, I was slipping deeper and deeper into depression. I just couldn't understand why this was happening to me and why everyone around me seemed to be getting pregnant with ease. Dilip and I started fighting a lot, but kept holding onto our dream of becoming parents. We moved onto IVF and while everything looked good with the treatment, the result was the same as the others; I had not become pregnant. After my second IVF resulted in all of my embryos arresting, I was told that I had poor egg quality. While I didn't believe this to be the case, I knew that I had had enough with the treatments and trying to have a biological baby.

We sent in our application to the adoption agency a few months after our IVF cycle, and found out that we were pregnant the same day that agency stamped our application. We were beyond excited at this news! While we didn't share our news with everyone, we announced to it to our close friends and immediate family. We saw the heartbeat on the ultrasound and were so happy that our struggle with infertility was finally over.

About 11 weeks into the pregnancy, I started getting cramps and spotting. I knew what was happening, but kept praying that it wasn't what I thought it was. I ended up in the emergency room and lost the baby on Mother's Day of all days. Dilip and I were completely devastated, but were not about to give up our dream of becoming parents. After we grieved this terrible loss, we got back to work on adopting a baby.

While all this was going on, I turned to my yoga and meditation practice daily to help me through the emotional ups and downs that I was going through. I started teaching Fertility Yoga and began leading a support group with RESOLVE, the national infertility organization. Without the support of the women in my group and classes, I'm not sure how I would have survived everything we went through.

Almost a year to the day that we lost our baby, we adopted our beautiful son, Raj. When I saw him for the first time, I knew that the healing had begun and that everything we went through was worth it. I continued to teach Fertility Yoga and lead the support group as I wanted nothing more than to help women who were going through what I had gone through.

It is my hope that this book will offer women some alternative and/or complementary practices as they try to fulfill their dreams of having a baby. I hope that this book will help you feel less isolated and alone if you are having trouble trying to conceive, as that was perhaps one of the most challenging aspects of my own personal journey. Finally, I hope that yoga teachers and others who are not personally trying to conceive may benefit from learning more about the process and how yoga can help prepare the body for the miracle of pregnancy and giving birth and the blessing of becoming a parent.

Namaste,
Jill Petigara

LYNN'S STORY

The table of contents for this book sat in the bottom drawer of my desk for over five years. That it is finally written is evidence to me of the truth of this quote by one of my teacher's teachers, the late Sufi master, Pir Vilayat Inayat Khan, "If you dedicate yourself to service, the doors will open." Not that I had purposefully planned to dedicate myself to service. It is just that my life kept moving away from what I had been doing for some years (international management) and moving toward teaching yoga, and specifically, teaching yoga for fertility.

I started doing yoga when I was living in Asia in the mid-1980s. When I returned to the states, it was to attend an MBA program at the University of Washington in Seattle. I continued my yoga practice through the stress of graduate school and as I started a career doing international management for high-tech companies.

As my career continued to advance, I took on responsibility for managing the international sales and marketing for a growing software company, which meant a lot of international travel. I was eventually managing a network of partners in over 40 countries, and a staff that spanned three continents. It was challenging, interesting, exciting, and exhausting. I became an expert in hotel room yoga, airport yoga, and even airplane yoga. I would rush from the airport, just off an 18-hour flight from Singapore, and head straight to yoga class.

In the midst of this, when I was in my early thirties, we decided that we should try to start a family. After trying for nearly two years, we went to a fertility clinic for a check-up. The doctor advised us that we were going to need to be in the same country at least during ovulation, or it wasn't ever going to work! I was also diagnosed with endometriosis, for which I underwent a six-month drug regimen, followed by a laparoscopic surgery. Neither of these treatments allowed us to achieve a pregnancy.

In retrospect, it is not at all surprising that I did not get pregnant. Working against it were the job stress, the international travel that constantly disrupted my sleep patterns and internal body rhythms, and a very real, although probably not quite conscious, concern about how I was going to work a newborn into my job schedule. After almost five years, and various other medical interventions, I finally started my own consulting business to get control over my travel schedule, and we decided to try IVF. I should probably have given myself time to really de-stress and replenish myself at this point (more on this in Chapter 8), but that is easier to say in hindsight!

We decided ahead of time that we would try up to three rounds of IVF, and after that would pursue adoption. After our first unsuccessful cycle, I had a very strong vision of an Asian-featured baby (neither of us have Asian heritage). Because of the strength of this vision, I began to feel that IVF might not be our path. Still, I agreed to go ahead with the next cycles as we had planned. My yoga practice really helped offset the added stress and added hormones of the IVF process. I noticed that I had fewer of the mood swings and side effects from the medications than others I knew who were going through IVF at the same time. I was disappointed, but not terribly surprised, when our last two IVF cycles also did not work.

We had just started moving forward with paperwork for the adoption process, when we got a call from one of the handful of people in the world who knew what we were doing. He wondered if we were ready to adopt, because he knew of some potential birth parents we might like to meet. "By the way," he said, "the birth father is Asian." "OH!" I yelled into the phone. "That IS our baby!" And so, only two months after we let go of our seven-year process of trying to conceive, my infant son was in my arms. And, this many years later, it is absolutely clear that he was the right child, and that he arrived at exactly the right time.

Our experience taught me a couple of essential things. First, it was a lesson in the importance of keeping a strong intention to be parents, but also the importance of not trying to control the details of how that happens. The Universe (or God, or Spirit, or whomever you believe is helping us) needs space to grant our wishes, because we ourselves may not know what the right path is. In the yogic tradition we are counseled to reserve our judgment about what is the "best" way for things to happen, because we are really not able to say, from our surface perspective, what is a "good" thing and what is a "bad" thing. Yogis believe that there is intrinsically good and bad in everything.

The second key thing I learned was the importance of believing in my own intuition. It happened several times during our fertility journey, where I was told things by people who were undisputed experts in their fields, but which didn't jive with what my own intuition said was true for me. For example, our highly experienced adoption attorney, who was an adoptive parent

himself, told us there was a "one in a thousand chance" that our adoption would go through, given what we had told him of the circumstances. In my heart, I knew he was wrong, but my mind bought into the fear that he might be right. This heart-mind conflict was the source of a lot of stress for a few weeks, until it became clear that my intuition was correct, and the adoption would, in fact, go through.

After the sleep-deprivation stage of babyhood was past, I decided I wanted to start a yoga program specifically for women who were trying to conceive. I realized how much I had benefitted from my own yoga practice during my long fertility journey. I also felt (again, in hindsight) that the yoga practice I had been doing had perhaps been more strenuous than was helpful. I began to research this, and developed the Yoga for Fertility program that I have been teaching through weekly classes, workshops and retreats since 2002. During this time, I was still running my international consulting business, but I found that when I walked into my office and saw the two different stacks of work, I would invariably be drawn to the pile that was yoga related. Thus, my yoga teaching began to grow, and my consulting business began to play second fiddle.

When I first started to think about writing a book on yoga for fertility, I had been teaching the yoga for fertility program for about five years. I wrote the table of contents, did some research, and then the doors began to open. One student's husband was a publisher and offered to help with my book proposal. Another student was a well-known personality and writer for *Time magazine*, *The Washington Post*, and other publications, and offered to help connect me with publishers. And yet, despite all the support, I didn't manage to get it written. At the time, in addition to my teaching schedule, I was trying to figure out how to help my son who was really struggling in school (we eventually learned he has dyslexia). I was just unable to devote the energy and time to the book project.

Then, at the beginning of 2011, I realized that I finally had the time and energy available to write the book, and that I really wanted to make it happen. So, I sat down and had a talk with the Universe. I apologized for wasting the resources it offered last time, and promised to go through with the project if it were at all possible to be given a second chance.

Shortly after that, I read an article in *The New York Times* about Yoga for Fertility, and noticed a quote from Jill Petigara, who was teaching fertility yoga near Philadelphia. A few weeks later, I saw that Jill had given a webcast talk on fertility yoga for RESOLVE, the national infertility organization. Since there were so few people teaching yoga for fertility, I was interested to talk with Jill, and we connected by phone. About three-quarters of an hour into the conversation, Jill said, "I feel funny asking you this, since we have never met, and I've only talked with you for 45 minutes, but would you be interested in writing a book with me?" I said, "Well, funny you should ask me that! I just happen to have a table of contents for a book on yoga for fertility sitting in my bottom drawer."

Jill had received a call from Noreen Henson, Executive Director of Demos Health Publishing, who had seen her quoted in *The New York Times*, and who was interested in publishing a book on yoga for fertility. Jill was very interested, but with the realities of a full-time job and a two-year-old son, realized she would not be able to do it alone. Thus began our long-distance collaboration on this book. I am extremely grateful to Jill for taking the risk of opening her project to someone else, especially someone she had never met (we did finally meet in person when Jill flew to Seattle for the photo shoot). I am also very grateful to the Universe for giving me a second chance—and this time, also including a co-author and a publisher in the deal, which was a pretty foolproof way to make sure it would happen this time!

From my personal experience as a long-time yoga practitioner and yoga teacher, I firmly believe that yoga benefits us in every aspect of our lives—physically, emotionally, mentally, and spiritually. I hope that the information in this book will help you on the path to parenthood in all of those ways. And, when you do become parents, I know that what you have learned in the process will help you to be the best possible parents, which is the most important job in the world!

Namaste,
Lynn Jensen

What Is Yoga for Fertility?

We are often asked the following questions about yoga for fertility:

- What is yoga for fertility?
- What are its benefits?
- How is it different from other types of yoga?
- Who can benefit from yoga for fertility?

This chapter will address those questions, starting with a look at how yoga can help with fertility. Even using the word "yoga" can imply different things to different people. To many people in the West, yoga means physical poses, or "asanas" that are taught to classes in gyms or yoga studios. Yoga is, in fact, not just physical poses, but a vast body of knowledge

that has developed over the past several thousand years, and that continues to develop. The word "yoga" means "union" or "yoke," which actually refers to the union between humans and the Divine, however the Divine is perceived. In this sense, we could think of yoga as a set of practices undertaken to get oneself more in tune with the Divine. Alternatively, we could think of yoga as a way to remove the barriers that separate us from the underlying energy field that powers the Universe.

This is a useful way to think of yoga when we talk about yoga for fertility. Creating new life is one of the basic themes of the universe. New stars, and even new galaxies, are created every day. Every species of plant and animal is driven to reproduce itself, in keeping with the laws of the universe. So, at the highest level, yoga for fertility is about learning to tune into those universal laws that govern creativity, fertility, and continuation of the species. The desire to create life is deeply embedded in the human soul. On a more physiological level, we can think of yoga practices as helping us "tune in" to the universal energy field, by reducing our reactivity to stresses, opening energy channels in the body, and calming the mind.

Over about the past fifty years, many different "brands" of yoga have cropped up in the West, which differentiate themselves by emphasizing different combinations of physical poses and sequences, or different approaches to teaching yoga poses. You may have heard of yoga studios offering descriptions of their classes in terms of "hot" yoga, or "power" yoga, or "flow" yoga. Or, you may be familiar with some varieties of yoga such as Ashtanga, Bikram, or Iyengar. But the inventors of these various "brands" are not generally thinking up new yoga poses or practices. Instead, they draw from the extensive repertoire of Hatha yoga poses that has been developed over hundreds, or even thousands of years. Yoga for fertility draws from this same repertoire. These poses and practices were developed to have specific effects on the human body—not only the physical body, but also the mental/emotional and spiritual "bodies."

Some General Yoga Benefits

- Increases flexibility and strength
- Improves balance and posture
- Maintains health of joints and spinal discs
- Increases circulation to all body systems, including organs
- Supports the lymphatic system, which is responsible for removal of toxins
- Regulates the endocrine system
- Boosts the immune system
- Improves sleep
- Reduces stress and calms the central nervous system
- Clears the brain; improves memory and the ability to concentrate
- Improves the efficiency and health of the respiratory system
- Increases oxygen to cells and increases red blood cell count
- Slows the aging process due to improved oxygenation of the blood, and detoxification of all systems
- Helps prevent osteoporosis by increasing strength. Yoga helps reduce cortisol levels in the blood stream, stemming the loss of calcium
- Increases overall energy level
- Improves metabolic efficiency, which helps with weight control
- Boosts libido and improves sexual performance
- Improves mood, reduces anxiety, and alleviates depression
- Reduces blood pressure and cholesterol levels

GENERAL YOGA BENEFITS

Yoga as a practice offers an incredible number of benefits to the practitioner. It builds muscular and bone strength, while also improving flexibility, posture and balance. Yoga poses such as twists help to keep joints and spinal discs lubricated, which keeps them working better, longer. Regular yoga practice supports virtually every system in the body, including the circulatory system, the respiratory system, the immune system, the endocrine system, the digestive system, the lymphatic system and the central nervous system. Yoga also helps to regulate bodily processes such as the cyclical rhythms responsible for our sleep/wake cycles, our monthly menstrual cycles, and our internal reactions to the seasons. There are also mental/emotional benefits, such as feelings of calm, non-reactivity to stressors, and mental clarity.

Long-term yoga practitioners usually look younger than they are, because of the constant revitalization that all of these systems receive. They also measure 5 to 10 years younger than their chronological age on physiological tests. From a fertility standpoint, this alone is a good reason to start a yoga practice.

This long list of yoga benefits has been documented by multiple studies, as well as medical practitioners' observations. One thing has become very clear: the more people who begin to practice yoga, the fewer health problems we will have as a population!

YOGA FOR FERTILITY BENEFITS

The benefits of yoga for fertility include those general benefits of yoga outlined above. What differentiates yoga for fertility as a practice is *which* poses and practices we choose to do, and sometimes, which we choose *not* to do. In yoga for fertility, we choose to focus on those poses and practices that specifically help us prepare for ovulation, conception and pregnancy.

The box below lists benefits which are all important aspects of a fertility yoga

Yoga for Fertility Benefits

1. Increases energy and blood flow, especially in the heart and pelvic areas
2. Stimulates the reproductive system directly by focusing on the ovaries and uterus
3. Supports and helps to regulate the endocrine (glandular/hormonal) system
4. Reduces levels of stress hormones in the bloodstream
5. Adapts poses according to the phase of the woman's monthly cycle
6. Calms the mind and reduces negative thinking
7. Opens a two-way communication channel between mind and body
8. Uses yoga, meditation, and visualization to help synchronize messages between the conscious mind, the subconscious mind, and the body
9. Balances feminine/masculine or yin/yang energy in the body
10. Increases "apana," or the downward-flowing energy in the body and "samana," the digestive and absorptive energy in the body
11. Builds life-force energy in the body

practice. In order to understand more about how these can help enhance fertility, let's look at each benefit in greater detail.

1. INCREASES ENERGY AND BLOOD FLOW

If we want the glands and organs of the pelvis (including the ovaries, uterus, and Fallopian tubes) to be healthy and functioning at their maximum effectiveness, we need to supply them with a continuous flow of nutrient- and oxygen-rich blood. While it is the job of the heart to keep blood pumping around the body, we can help or hinder the heart in its mission to get fresh blood to all parts of the body. If we are holding a lot of tension in the pelvis, the blood vessels can become constricted, cutting down the flow to key organs. If we spend a large part of our day sitting, the blood can tend to stagnate in the pelvic area, thus "starving" the pelvic organs of the nutrients they should be receiving from a continuously refreshed blood flow.

Energy flow, while perhaps not as obvious as blood flow, is equally important from the yogic point of view. If energy flow is a new concept to you, it may help to think of having an energy system, similar to the circulatory system, in our bodies. In the yoga tradition, the vessels or channels in this system are called "nadis." This is similar to the concept of "chi" in Chinese medicine. The nadis serve to move fresh energy to all parts of the body, similar to the way that arteries move fresh blood. In our discussion of potentially tension-holding spots such as the pelvis and heart areas, we can imagine that anything that restricts the flow of blood may also restrict the flow of energy to a particular area.

Surprisingly, the pelvis is one of the key tension-holding areas in the body, although we rarely notice it as much as we might notice tension in the shoulders or neck. We can end up with pelvic tension for different reasons. Sometimes it results from physical exercise such as running, walking, hiking, soccer, biking, or other exercise that strengthens but also tightens the pelvic muscles. Sometimes we hold tension in the pelvis that has to do with a previous life trauma centered in the pelvis, such as sexual abuse, past abortions or miscarriages, injuries or diseases. In yoga, we regard the pelvis as not only the center of reproduction, but also as the center of creative endeavors of any sort. So, we could be holding tension in the pelvis as a result of being unable to express ourselves creatively in our lives. Tami Lynn Kent, in her book "Wild Feminine" says essentially that we stuff lots of things that are difficult to deal with in the pelvic area.[1] Whatever the reason for the pelvic tension, releasing that tension is one of the important benefits of yoga for fertility.

The need for blood and energy to move through the heart area may seem less clearly related to fertility, at least from the Western point of view, which tends to compartmentalize the body. However, from the Eastern point of view, the heart area is very much related to the ability to conceive. One of the key tenets of fertility from the Chinese medicine point of view is that the "heart-to-uterus energy channel" must be open in order for conception to occur. In the same way that the pelvic area can hold tension, the heart area (often referred to as the "heart center" or the "heart chakra" in yoga) can become tight and closed, restricting the flow of blood and energy.

What causes this closing down of the heart center? Once again, the culprit can be physical practices or emotional stresses. Physically, our posture and our daily activities can impact the heart center. If we spend much of our day hunched over a computer or a steering wheel, we are likely to be rounding forward and physically collapsing the heart center. Emotional stresses on the heart can include any experience where we feel betrayed or where we have suffered a loss. Dealing with fertility challenges can certainly stress the heart as we suffer a loss of our dream of pregnancy month after month. In addition, we sometimes feel as though our body has betrayed us by not doing what we always expected it to be able to do. Opening the heart center to increased blood and energy flow is another important benefit of yoga for fertility.

2. STIMULATES THE REPRODUCTIVE SYSTEM

In fertility yoga routines, we choose yoga poses which have the specific effect of bringing extra blood flow to the abdominal area, providing additional stimulation for the ovaries, uterus, and other abdominal organs. Some of these poses, such as legs-up-the-wall pose, provide this stimulation by positioning the body so that extra blood flows to the abdominal area. Other poses, such as locust pose, provide alternating compression and release to the low belly area. The result is that during the compression part of the pose, organs are compressed and old blood is squeezed out. During the release, the organs and glands in the low belly get a fresh, new supply of blood, flooding them with more oxygen and nutrients. These are a few examples of how we can use particular yoga poses to direct more blood flow to a specific area of the body.

3. SUPPORTS AND REGULATES THE ENDOCRINE SYSTEM

The endocrine system includes all of the glands in the body. The proper functioning of the endocrine system is absolutely critical to fertility. Scientists and doctors are continually discovering additional ways in which the endocrine system impacts and controls key aspects of the reproductive process. A few glands, such as the ovaries and thyroid gland, have for a long time been clearly implicated in fertility problems. If they are not working properly, the ovaries may not be ovulating at the right time, or may not be ovulating at all. If the thyroid gland is either a tiny bit underactive or overactive, fertility suffers. In fact, if any gland in the endocrine system is out of balance, it can have a negative impact on fertility. One of our key goals in yoga for fertility is to help regulate the endocrine system so that each gland is working as effectively and efficiently as possible.

Fortunately for us, yoga is innately designed to work on the endocrine system. If you superimpose a map of the endocrine system onto a map of the key yogic energy centers (called chakras), you will find that they line up nicely. Although yoga was developed long before the endocrine system was described by Western medicine, it was designed to work on the chakras, which the sages perceived to be very important energy centers in the body. Western medicine has since confirmed this by furthering our understanding of the important role the endocrine system plays in all aspects of health.

The good news is that every yoga pose we do in any yoga class is working on at least one or more of the glands in the endocrine system. In yoga for fertility, we may choose poses that target specific glands, such as the ovaries, thyroid, or adrenal glands in order to specifically support regulation of those glands.

4. REDUCES STRESS HORMONE LEVELS

One of the most widely recognized benefits of yoga is its role in stress reduction. Numerous studies have shown it to be effective in reducing stress in a broad range of populations, such as in cancer patients and veterans with post-traumatic stress disorder. There is no question that ongoing fertility challenges are stress-producing. A famous study by Dr. Alice Domar at the Harvard Medical School documented that the anxiety and depression levels of women facing fertility challenges was on par with the levels of people who had been diagnosed with terminal diseases.[2]

Stress, whether due to our jobs, our relationships, our life situations, or fertility challenges, can negatively impact our ability to become pregnant. When we are under stress, our adrenal glands pump so-called "stress hormones," such as adrenaline and cortisol, into our bloodstream. The role of these hormones is to activate the sympathetic nervous system. This starts certain physiological changes happening in the body, which are supposed to prepare us to deal with the stressful situation.

This combination of physiological responses has been called "the fight-or-flight response." The adrenal glands are supposed to react to short-term danger by preparing the body to either fight or take flight, and they do a good job of this. All of these physiological changes would be very useful if we were being attacked by a saber-tooth tiger! However, when we are under continuous stress, the adrenal glands continue to pump out stress hormones, hour after hour. Now, the physiological changes are not so helpful. Particularly if we are trying to get pregnant, we do NOT want the blood flow to the core organs restricted, nor do we want shallow breathing. We are robbing the uterus and ovaries of the rich blood flow and oxygen they require to function optimally.

Physiological Changes Associated with the "Fight-or-Flight" Response

- Breathing becomes shallower and more rapid
- Blood vessels in the core of the body restrict
- Heart beats rapidly, rushing blood to the arms and legs
- Blood pressure increases
- Muscles tense
- Adrenal glands secrete stress hormones such as cortisol and adrenaline
- Brain goes on hyper-alert
- Hypothalamus releases endorphins, which are the body's natural pain-killers
- Immune system is depressed
- Digestive system shuts down

Recalibrating the body's reaction to stress is one of our key goals in yoga for fertility. While we may not be able to remove all the stressors from our lives, we can effectively reduce our reaction to stress events. This, in turn, will minimize stress hormone levels in the bloodstream. We can do this by eliciting the "relaxation response," a term coined by cardiologist Dr. Herbert Benson in the late 1960s. Yoga and meditation are particularly effective in eliciting the relaxation response. They activate the parasympathetic nervous system, allowing the body to reverse the physiological effects of the fight-or-flight response, and instead activating the relaxation response. Interestingly, the hypothalamus gland, which mediates the relaxation response, also regulates all aspects of reproduction.[3]

Physiological Changes Associated with the Relaxation Response

- Heart rate decreases
- Blood pressure lowers
- Breathing rate slows
- Oxygen consumption decreases
- Level of stress hormones in blood stream drops
- Reduction in muscle tension and constriction
- Blood returns to core organs
- Changes brainwaves to calmer, slower patterns

In our experience with the women in our classes, the relaxation aspect of yoga alone is extremely important. Most of our students are busy career women with demanding jobs. Usually, a few students in each class already have a child at home, and are now working as well as being a mother, while trying to conceive again. Having a time set aside to just focus on themselves, where they can relax deeply, is so valuable.

A few years ago, at the end of the initial class in a new session, one of the students came up to me with tears in her eyes, and said, "I didn't realize until now that I really have not relaxed for at least the past year. Thank you!"

5. ADAPTS POSES ACCORDING TO THE MONTHLY CYCLE

The function of each portion of a woman's monthly cycle is specific to that part of the cycle. So, in yoga for fertility we tailor the poses accordingly. In the first half of the cycle leading up to ovulation, the most important focus is on stimulating the ovaries to produce follicles and release a high-quality egg. We would also like to ensure that the uterus is developing a thick, lush lining. So, in the first half of the cycle, we choose yoga poses which bring stimulation to the area of the ovaries and improve blood flow to the uterus. In the second half of the cycle, post-ovulation, we are interested in supporting implantation. Thus, we choose yoga poses that are a bit less stimulating, and more supportive and calming. During menstruation, our main objective is to rest the body and support the movement of blood out of the uterus.

This is one of the reasons that we suggest following the yoga for fertility routines if you are trying to conceive, even if you are already doing a regular yoga practice. It is best to tailor the routine to where you are in your cycle. Other considerations for your practice, if you are attending another yoga class, are discussed in Chapter 6.

6. CALMS THE MIND AND REDUCES NEGATIVE THINKING

One of the concepts we teach in yoga for fertility classes is the practice of having *both* the body and the mind present during yoga practice. We ask our students to try to "be present" in the yoga class. This is essentially just practice focusing on what we are doing; i.e., to have the body and mind engaged in the same thing at the same time. This may sound like an unusual thing to practice, but the truth is that we rarely have our mind fully present with what our body is doing.

Think of the last time you drove to the grocery store. Were you thinking "Here I am, sitting in the car with my hands on the steering wheel?" Unlikely! Your mind was probably already at your destination, figuring out what you needed to buy, and possibly even thinking about what you were going to do after you finished shopping!

Yet, there are some very good reasons to cultivate having the mind and body in the same place at the same time. Of course, one reason is that you will probably do a better job of what you are doing (like driving!) if you are actually thinking about it. But from the fertility perspective, the most important reason is that it reduces stress. Most of our stress does not come from what is happening right at this moment. Ninety-eight percent of the time our stress comes from things that happened in the past, or things that we are afraid might happen in the future.

In yoga, we talk about the "monkey mind" that runs around back and forth. It pulls things from the past to stress over, and from the future to worry about, and generally gets into mischief. It often tries to drag you back to the same stressful scenario over and over. Being present helps to control the "monkey mind," but it takes practice. You may want to start by trying to

---

Study Finds Happiness Linked to Where the Mind Is

A pair of Harvard psychologists recently carried out a study on happiness. The study used a smartphone application to check in with a number of individuals at various times during the day, over a period of a few weeks. Each time, the individuals were asked to respond to several questions, such as:

1. What are you doing?
2. What are you thinking about?
3. How are you feeling?

At the end of the study, the researchers compiled the responses. The study found that 47% of the time, people were thinking about something other than what they were doing. The researchers concluded that a main cause of people's unhappiness is how frequently their minds wander. What they found was that the people who reported feeling happiest were those who were *thinking about what they were doing*. These people were even happier than those who were thinking about some positive thing, like being on the beach in Hawaii![4]

---

stay present in your yoga practice as you do the routines in this book. Do not be discouraged if your own "monkey mind" runs off somewhere else every few minutes or even every few seconds. Usually the "monkey mind" has had a lot of practice getting into trouble, and does not take kindly to being brought under control!

7. TWO-WAY COMMUNICATION BETWEEN MIND AND BODY

One big advantage of being present in your yoga practice is that it makes it possible to get messages and feedback from the body to the brain. In other words, it allows information from the body to be brought to your conscious awareness. The requirement for this, of course, is that your brain is paying attention to what your body is doing. Unfortunately, our mind-body communication channel often works only in one direction: mind-to-body. Our minds are used to telling the body what to do, and having the body obey without complaint.

For example, imagine you are sitting at your computer working on a report that is due tomorrow morning. Your neck and shoulders say, "Ouch, this is too long in this position! Please get up and stretch! We are hurting!" But what is your response? It is likely that you ignore this message altogether, because you have a report that needs to be finished. If you were to tune into the body and really use two-way mind-body communication, you would probably get up and stretch. And you would likely find that your brain worked better after you stretched, since you released the blockages to the blood flowing into the brain. Thus, you would be more efficient in finishing your report.

8. SYNCHRONIZES THE MESSAGES BETWEEN THE CONSCIOUS MIND, THE SUBCONSCIOUS MIND, AND THE BODY

Yoga helps us access wisdom and information that resides in the body that we may be aware of on a subconscious level, but that our conscious mind has not noticed. This is particularly important in yoga for fertility. During the process of trying to conceive, we are often required to notice what is happening in our bodies and make decisions based on that information. Am I about to ovulate? Am I feeling different than I did last month? Is my period on the way? How is this medication affecting me? Is this a good month for us to try, or to take a break? The more we are able to tune into our body's messages, the more likely it is that we will make appropriate and effective decisions.

9. BALANCES ENERGY IN THE BODY

According to Eastern philosophy, everyone is made up of a combination of feminine and masculine energy. Ideally, the two are at an optimum ratio and balance each other, although people with perfectly balanced energy are exceedingly rare. A graphic representation of this concept of opposite energies balancing is the ancient Chinese symbol for Yin (feminine) and Yang (masculine).

The Yang (masculine) energy is considered to be the more action-oriented, "hot" energy, and is also represented by the sun. The Yin (feminine) energy is the more intuitive, contemplative, "cool" energy, and is considered to be the "moon"

The Yin/Yang Symbol Representing Balance of Opposites

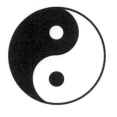

energy. The word "hatha," as in "hatha yoga" also reflects these two opposite energies in balance. "Ha" refers to the energy of the sun, and "tha" to the energy of the moon. Further, the yogic understanding of the energy system in the body is that there are three major energy channels which carry energy from the base of the spine up to the crown of the head, and beyond. The Ida channel carries the male (Yang) energy, and the Pingala channel carries the female (Yin) energy. These channels wind around in a spiral, with the third channel, the Susumna, in the center of the spiral. In fact, the concept of balancing male and female energies is of central importance in many Eastern practices. If the male (Yang) energy gets too strong, we find a person who is all action, doing without thinking deeply. If the female (Yin) energy is stronger, we may find a person who is very thoughtful, but unable to take action when needed. To optimize fertility, the ideal condition would be to have the Yin and Yang energies perfectly balanced in the body. This is a state of calm, where the tension between the two has come into equilibrium.

Generally, we see that most of the women who come to our classes have an imbalance, with the Yang being too strong. The likely reason for this is that our culture

in the United States tends to be very Yang-oriented. Undoubtedly, there are some jobs that are more Yin-enhancing, such as working with children, artistic professions, or some types of health care or teaching jobs. But mostly, it is the take-action, "just do it" philosophy that is rewarded and encouraged in our culture, as opposed to the contemplative mode. Many of us are in jobs or careers with an overwhelming workload, where we have to take lots of actions quickly. Even driving to work, if we happen to live in a city and need to take the freeway, can raise our Yang energy. By the time we get to yoga for fertility class, we are in need of some balancing of that Yang energy. This is one of the key reasons behind the poses we choose to do in yoga for fertility class.

Within the overall body of hatha yoga poses, there are yoga poses that are more Yang-enhancing, and poses that are more Yin-enhancing. In a balanced yoga practice, one would choose some Yang poses and some Yin poses, with the idea that these would balance each other out. The end result would be that the practitioner is left with a calm, centered energy after the practice. Many of the most popular "brands" of yoga in the United States today are very Yang-intensive practices. They are using primarily poses which strengthen and heat the body. The poses may be done quickly, one after the other, in a "flow" style, without any rest between poses. In addition, some classes may be conducted in heated rooms, which further adds to the Yang energy generated by the practice.

If you have been practicing this type of yoga, you may find yoga for fertility routines to be not very "challenging." There is a reason for this. Our goal in yoga for fertility is not so much to strengthen the body, as to strengthen the central nervous system. We want to train the body to cope better with stress. We want to supply the organs and glands with more blood flow and oxygen, rather than rob them to supply the extremities for an intensive yoga practice. We want to bring up the Yin energy in the body, as this is the energy that is more conducive to conception and motherhood.

TYPES OF YOGA AND THEIR USEFULNESS FOR FERTILITY SUPPORT	
Generally supportive of fertility	**Less supportive of fertility**
Yoga for fertility	Hot yoga
Gentle yoga	Power yoga
Restorative yoga	Any yoga in heated room
Yoga nidra	Intensive, heat-producing practices
	Flow or vinyasa yoga

Notes:

1. In order to make these lists, we had to generalize based on what we have observed being done in "standard" classes of the various types. There may be, for example, some gentle yoga classes that are not so great for fertility, and some flow yoga classes that do many supportive fertility poses. And this is not to say that one cannot get pregnant doing the yoga practices in Column 2. But on the whole, we would recommend yoga classes in Column 1, before those in Column 2, for anyone trying to conceive.
2. There is a type of yoga called "Yin Yoga," which you may have heard of; however, the philosophy of this type of yoga is different than what we are talking about here with focus on a Yin practice.
3. In Chapter 6, we will talk about some basic ways you can modify your practice if you are attending another yoga class, to make it more "fertility friendly."

10. INCREASES APANA AND SAMANA

The yoga picture of the body recognizes five energy currents that represent the flow of life-force energies. Two of these currents, the apana and samana, are especially important to support fertility. Apana helps with elimination, and as such supports a healthy menstrual cycle. It also aids in the removal of toxins, which could impact fertility if stuck in the body. Samana supports the digestive and respiratory processes so that our bodies can make efficient use of the food we eat and the air we breathe to nourish our bodies. Specific yoga poses increase apana and samana, and these poses are included in the yoga for fertility routines we offer in the following chapters.

11. BUILDS LIFE-FORCE ENERGY (PRANA) IN THE BODY

Yoga recognizes prana as the spark of life, the vitality that permeates all the cells of the body and essentially makes us alive. You might think about prana like the charge in a battery. When it runs down, our bodies, our health, and even our emotional lives don't work so well. The quantity of prana that we have impacts the quality of our lives and our health. Prana is very important for conception. It makes sense that, in order to create new life, we need to have a good store of life-force energy to begin with.

Unfortunately, our modern lifestyles tend to drain us of prana, rather than build it. Many times we are in a "prana-deficit" when we decide to try to conceive. Things that drain prana include general stress, a cluttered, chaotic living or working environment, negative people, traffic, pollution, poor diet, overly strenuous exercise, job stress, relationships, etc. In fact, many of the things that we may have to deal with on a daily basis can deplete our stores of prana. A regular, daily yoga for fertility practice is a good way to replenish and increase prana. The practice of hatha yoga postures, pranayama (yogic breathing techniques) and the use of mantras, meditation, and visualization all help to build more of this life-force energy. Other ways you can build prana include eating whole, non-processed, nutritious foods, taking a long walk in nature, or singing, chanting or meditating.

2

Who Can Benefit from Yoga for Fertility?

JUST STARTING OUT

Over the years we have been teaching yoga for fertility, we have worked with over a thousand women and couples who are trying to conceive. In our experience, yoga can help with fertility in a whole range of conditions. If you are just starting to try to conceive, yoga for fertility will help prepare the entire endocrine and reproductive systems to be working as effectively as possible. The earlier you start, the better, as yoga has a cumulative effect over time.

UNEXPLAINED INFERTILITY

If you have been diagnosed with "unexplained infertility," you are not alone. This is a rather common diagnosis, and hints at the fact that current science and medicine does not yet understand, or have the ability to address, many of the factors that impact fertility. In these cases, yoga can help unravel the factors that may be contributing to the fertility issues. Imbalances in the hormonal system, which have not been detected because they lie outside the normal fertility clinic testing, may be responsible. As we have seen, yoga can help support the endocrine system, and over time will help to regulate some of these imbalances.

Another common contributing factor to unexplained infertility can be the body's response to high stress levels, which causes non-fertility-supporting physiological changes in the body. Yoga has been clearly shown to help to calm the body's fight-or-flight reaction, and reverse those physiological changes.

A third common factor in unexplained infertility can be emotional or subconcious barriers to conception. The nature of yoga is that it helps peel away the layers of "avidya," which we regard in yoga as matter that clouds our clear perception of things. The Western version of "avidya" might be layers of emotional patterning. These layers create obstacles to our being able to see situations clearly, and accomplish what we are intrinsically completely capable of doing. Mind/body medicine continues to demonstrate how innately linked the body's responses are to our emotional states. Yoga helps to balance our emotional responses.

PCOS

An increasingly common diagnosis we see in women with fertility challenges is polycystic ovarian syndrome (PCOS). This is a condition in which the ovaries produce many small, cyst-like follicles, which fail to develop properly. It is attributed to an insulin/blood sugar imbalance in the bloodstream—a condition that is controlled by the pancreas. The pancreas is one of the glands in the endocrine system, which sits near the kidneys and adrenal glands. As

we have seen, yoga for fertility can help to rebalance the endocrine system, and thus can be helpful in improving the underlying conditions that cause PCOS.

ENDOMETRIOSIS

Another fairly common diagnosis for fertility issues is endometriosis, a condition in which cells like those that line the uterus (the endometrium) attach to other tissues inside the abdomen. An estimated five to seven million American women currently suffer from endometriosis, according to the *Journal of the American Medical Association*. About 40% of women with infertility may have some level of endometriosis.

It is not usually possible to give a definitive diagnosis of endometriosis without actually looking into the abdominal cavity, although ultrasounds can sometimes indicate its presence. A laparoscope is used to see into the pelvic cavity to look for the lesions that indicate endometriosis, and sometimes these are removed surgically. Endometriosis lesions can be found on the uterus, ovaries, Fallopian tubes, and even in areas of the body far from the pelvis, such as the lungs. Sometimes the lesions can bind the reproductive organs to the pelvic walls or ligaments, or other organs. Endometriosis may be exacerbated by excess estrogen.

There is no real consensus about the cause or the cure for endometriosis. There have been some studies suggesting that reducing general inflammation in the body can help alleviate endometriosis.[1] Dietary changes, supplementing with antioxidants, yoga, and stress reduction techniques can all help reduce inflammation.

We have observed that gentle yoga can help alleviate the discomfort of endometriosis, which often causes debilitating pain. Also, if excess estrogen is contributing to the problem, yoga for fertility can help rebalance the hormonal system to correct the estrogen/progesterone ratio.

MISCARRIAGE

Over the years, we have had many women in our yoga for fertility classes who have had one or more miscarriages. We have found it to be the case almost universally that these women eventually are able to carry a pregnancy to term. Sometimes, in addition to adding a daily yoga practice, this has required making some lifestyle or dietary changes, or dealing with some emotional or other factors. In some percentage of cases, medical intervention is also required.

Continuing a yoga practice has helped them cope with the stress of miscarriage, as well as helping to overcome the underlying problems that may have contributed to the pregnancy losses. Yoga for fertility classes can also offer a support system for women grieving from miscarriage. Usually in our classes there are a few women who have been through miscarriages, and so the level of understanding and empathy is very high. In our culture, this type of support system is otherwise very much lacking. Often, women who have had miscarriages are just expected to carry on, or try again, without any acknowledgment of their deep and recent losses. Sometimes, accumulated grief from miscarriages can impede further attempts to conceive. Because yoga helps to move emotional energy rather than allowing it to just sit and accumulate, yoga is a useful tool for working with grief, as well as other strong emotions.

Indira's Story from Lynn's Yoga for Fertility Class

Several years ago, Indira joined one of my yoga for fertility classes. Although she had been born in India, she had not done yoga before. In fact, she told me that her mother and her mother's friends used to do yoga at her house, and her mother would try to get her to join them. But she thought yoga was silly and old-fashioned, and refused to try it. She was a modern Indian woman, who worked in a high-stress job as a project manager in a high-tech company.

From the start, I could see that Indira lived almost totally "in her head." Her body awareness was so poor that she was unable to follow my instructions in class. She simply had no idea what her body was doing (or not doing). Not only was two-way mind/body communication missing, but even one-way communication from the mind to the body was lacking. Her fertility history included six miscarriages over the past two years. It is perhaps not surprising that she had decided to "ex-communicate" her body!

Indira soon realized that yoga was helping her feel less stress in her daily life, and told me she thought that maybe her mother had been right about yoga! She checked out yoga books from the library, and would stay after class to ask me questions that had come up while she was reading them. It was not surprising to me that she chose such an academic, head-centered approach to learning yoga, as it seemed to be the way she approached

(*continued*)

everything in her life. But she also began to practice yoga at home for at least an hour a day using a routine I prepared for her. She was very disciplined, and she practiced yoga every day for over a year. Over this time, I noticed a big change in her ability to pay attention to her body while in yoga class.

When she got pregnant again, she was understandably very nervous after having endured so many miscarriages. Her husband was so concerned that he refused to let her drive, and instead he brought her to class every week and waited for her outside. She continued her home yoga practice with a modified routine for early pregnancy. She passed the eight-week mark, which had been the point of her previous miscarriages, and was feeling fine. By the end of the first trimester, she began to believe that this pregnancy could stick. It did, and she now has a very healthy son.

Indira has continued to practice yoga at home in the ensuing years, as she has become convinced of what her mother was trying to tell her so many years ago. Yoga helped her achieve her and her husband's dreams of parenthood. It has also helped her understand and believe in the wisdom of her body.

IS YOGA FOR FERTILITY HELPFUL FOR MEN?

The short answer to this question is "yes, absolutely." While hormone imbalances are not as big an issue for men as for women, men often have other impediments to fertility that yoga can help with. For instance, men who have desk jobs often suffer from stagnation in the pelvic/reproductive area, just as women do. Yoga helps to increase circulation and energy in the pelvic region. And men may be even more inclined to "stuff" their emotions, particularly their reactions to fertility challenges. Yoga can help them move through these emotions, and men are often more comfortable moving than talking. In addition, many men are working in stressful jobs, so a stress-reduction program is equally valuable for them.

While the information in this book more specifically addresses women's fertility challenges, it is important to remember that at least 25% of fertility challenges are due to male factor specifically, and for a full 50%, the male is a contributing factor. And yet, most treatment programs focus on the woman. The basic yoga routines we offer in this book are also helpful for men. We would strongly suggest, when possible, that couples practice yoga for fertility together. We have had many couples attend our yoga for fertility workshops, or take private instruction together.

There are many benefits of doing yoga with your partner/spouse. For one, it is just easier to keep up with the discipline of doing a daily practice if your significant other is doing it with you. Partners can also assist each other with some of the poses, increasing the benefit of the poses.

When dealing with fertility challenges, or when trying to conceive becomes paramount, a couple's sex life often suffers. Spontaneity may go out of the window and the need to perform "on demand" can dampen desire. Yoga offers a non-sexual way to be together physically, which can bring back some of the intimacy that may get lost in the process of chasing conception.

A not-much-advertised benefit of yoga, but one that is well-known among regular practitioners, is that a daily yoga practice improves one's sex life. Several factors are responsible for this, including improved blood and energy flow to the reproductive organs, increased control, and better ability to "be present" with your partner during sex. Specific practices such as pelvic floor exercises, breathing practices, and legs-up-the-wall pose, are especially beneficial.

THE RESEARCH: IS YOGA FOR FERTILITY EFFECTIVE?

The most famous studies tying yoga and meditation to fertility have been done by Dr. Alice Domar at the Mind/Body Institute at Harvard Medical Center. In her studies, "infertile" women were assigned either to a control group, or to a group who participated in peer-support discussions, or to a group that received training in mind/body techniques such as yoga and meditation. Her studies showed that the women who practiced mind/body techniques achieved pregnancies at a rate *almost three times* that of the control group. Within the year following the program, 55% of the mind/body group became pregnant, compared to only 20% of the control group. In addition, 42% of the mind/body group's pregnancies were conceived naturally, compared to 20% of the control group.[2]

Although I haven't (yet) done a statistical analysis, I estimate that more than 80% of the women who start *and continue* in my classes eventually conceive. The average length of time a woman is enrolled in my classes is around twelve months. Doing a regular yoga practice at home definitely helps reduce the time it takes for the yoga to be effective.

For some women it takes longer, and some women decide to move the process along by using IVF or donor eggs. A majority of the women in my classes also use complementary treatments such as acupuncture, Chinese herbs, or abdominal massage. But my experience is that for women who commit to a gentle and supportive yoga program, like the yoga for fertility program, most will eventually be able to conceive either naturally or with assistance. And it is worth noting that most of the women who join my classes are not the "easy" fertility cases. They have generally already been trying to conceive for at least a year, and have very often already consulted a doctor or a fertility clinic about their situation. Their age range is generally between 33–45, with the average age around 38.

3

Getting Started with Yoga for Fertility

Congratulations on taking the first steps toward learning about yoga and fertility! If you've read Chapter 1, you already know how yoga can help improve your fertility and overall well-being. If you have never taken a yoga class before, this book will help you learn how to use yoga to help enhance your fertility while learning how to safely come in and out of the poses and cultivate greater mind-body awareness. The basic routines in Chapters 4 and 5 were developed to be used by yoga practitioners, as well as by people with little to no experience with yoga. Please read through the yoga sequences carefully before beginning a routine. The pictures are there to help you see what

the basic form should look like. Keep in mind that the models in the photos are seasoned yoga practitioners, so your poses may not look exactly the way they do in the book.

This book is organized around your monthly cycle, so there are chapters that are dedicated to helping you understand what is happening in your body and what yoga practice would be most beneficial during that time. **Chapter 4** provides both a basic and intermediate yoga routine for the first half of your cycle. These routines are best performed after the heaviest flow days of your period are finished, up until ovulation. The yoga poses in this chapter are designed to help stimulate the ovaries, as well as provide more blood flow to the pelvic region. **Chapter 5** provides both a basic and intermediate yoga routine for the second half of your cycle. These routines are best performed after ovulation up until the start of your period, if you have not conceived. These poses are also designed to provide more blood flow to the pelvic region and to help thicken the lining of the uterus for implantation. These poses are more calming and less stimulating than the first half poses, and are also safe to practice if conception has occurred. **Chapter 6** provides yoga routines that can be used for other conditions like when you are menstruating, early pregnancy, and a stress relieving practice that can also be used during an ART cycle. **Chapter 7** explores more practices to support your fertility such as meditation, visualizations, affirmations, and mantras. **Chapter 8** looks at how lifestyle changes can impact your fertility, while **Chapter 9** explores other complementary practices like acupuncture and fertility abdominal massage. **Chapter 9** also gives you information on using yoga with ART (assisted reproductive technology) and advice on how to discuss your situation with friends and family. **Chapter 10** provides case studies of women who have used yoga for fertility to help them achieve their goal of becoming a mother. We encourage you to thoroughly read this getting started chapter before moving ahead to the yoga routines. However, this book is not necessarily linear, so feel free to skip around and read what piques your interest the most.

GETTING STARTED

Before you begin the yoga routines in Chapters 4, 5 and 6, make sure you have considered the following:

1. You have a quiet space in your home where you can fit a standard size yoga mat which is 24" by 68" inches. Hardwood floors are great but low pile carpet works fine too.

2. You have a wall that is free of pictures, heaters or any other obstructions that you can use to help balance and use for **Legs Up the Wall** pose.

3. You might want to play some relaxing music during your yoga routine. Remember to turn off your phone so you are not interrupted during this time.

4. Recommended additional equipment: yoga strap (or a scarf), yoga block, wool or cotton blanket. Optional equipment: bolster (or a cushion, pillows, or extra blankets), eye pillow (a scarf or article of clothing can also be used to cover eyes).

5. You have not eaten a heavy meal within the past 2 hours. Light food like fruit or granola can be fine within an hour of class, but it is best to practice on an empty stomach.

6. You are wearing loose comfortable clothing including yoga or fitness apparel that is stretchy, not tight or restrictive.

7. You have nothing on your feet. Socks can be worn while practicing the restorative poses, but it's best to practice yoga in bare feet.

8. You do not have any medical conditions for which yoga practice is contraindicated. You are advised to check with your physician if you are unsure whether it is safe for you to do the yoga routines in this book.

9. You have read through this chapter so you know where you are in your cycle and know which routines are best suited to you.

10. You have committed to taking whatever time you have to be completely present with yourself and your practice. Even if you only have 10 minutes, dedicate this time to nurturing yourself through yoga.

DECIDING WHERE TO BEGIN IN THIS BOOK

The yoga routines in Chapters 4, and 5 are organized around your menstrual cycle. If you have your period, you should consult the yoga routine in Chapter 6. If you are toward the end of your period and have not yet ovulated, you should practice the basic yoga routine in Chapter 4. Many of the poses in this chapter are meant to help stimulate the ovaries to help optimize ovulation. If you are not sure if you have ovulated yet, take a look at the box below for help in determining when you are ovulating. If you are still not sure of the exact time you ovulate, just use your best judgment. The yoga sequences in each chapter are all fertility enhancing poses, so it's fine if you are a little off with the timing. The most cautious approach would be to choose the second half routines if you are not sure where you are in your cycle, or if you think you may have ovulated already.

If you have already ovulated and are in the two-week wait, it is best to perform the basic yoga routine found in Chapter 5. The poses in this routine are focused on increasing blood flow to the pelvic area and thickening the lining of the uterus. These poses also have more of a Yin (calming/passive) quality to them, so they are perfect for this time in your cycle.

We recommend that you start with the basic routines even if you have been practicing yoga for a while. The basic routines are a great introduction to fertility yoga, so it's a good idea to practice those routines first, before moving on to the intermediate routines.

How to Tell if You are Ovulating

1. **Consult the calendar.** A typical cycle lasts approximately 28 days, and we usually ovulate right in the middle of the cycle, so in the case of a 28-day cycle that would be at around Day 14. Your cycle may vary from 28 days, however, so the best way to know your fertile days is to use one of the methods below.
2. **Chart your temperature.** Keep track of your BBT (basal body temperature) using a basal body thermometer. Your basal body temperature is taken first thing in the morning before you have gotten out of bed. When you keep track of your BBT for a couple of months, you will begin to see patterns that can help you determine ovulation. After ovulation, you will see a rise in your BBT that stays steady until your period. The day before your body temperature rises would be the day that you are ovulating.

(continued)

3. **Pay attention to your body.** If you are like 20% of women, you may get a slight cramp in the lower abdominal area on one side when are ovulating. This cramping is referred to as mittelschmerz, which is German for "middle pain." This slight pain or series of cramps is thought to be caused by the release of the mature egg from the ovary during ovulation.

4. **Check your cervical mucus.** There is a change in the consistency and appearance of your cervical fluid leading up to ovulation. Cervical mucus becomes slippery and stretchy, with a consistency similar to raw egg white just before ovulation, so it can carry the sperm to the ovum. (For more information on this, see No. 6 below.)

5. **Buy an ovulation predictor kit.** Ovulation predictor kits will check your levels of LH (luteinizing hormone) and tell you the best 12 to 24 hours to try to conceive.

6. **Get a copy of *Taking Charge of Your Fertility*** by Toni Weschler. This is a very comprehensive and detailed reference book that can help you learn about your cycles, determine ovulation timing, and even point out irregularities in timing that may be impacting your fertility.[1]

HOW MUCH TIME AND HOW OFTEN SHOULD YOU DO THESE ROUTINES?

Each of the yoga routines in this book is designed to take between 30 and 40 minutes, depending on how long you stay in each pose. We do make recommendations for the number of breaths you should take in each pose, but the time it takes you to take those breaths is really quite individual. The breaths should be slow and deep, and you can decide how long you want to stay in each pose. If you do not have 30 to 40 minutes to dedicate to your practice every day, choose one pose like **Legs Up the Wall** and stay in it for 5 or 10 minutes rather than doing nothing at all. Any time of day is fine to practice, but try to get into a consistent routine if possible. Yoga does have a cumulative effect on the body, so the more you do it, the better, but don't allow this to be another thing you have to add to your To Do List. If you can dedicate three times a week to the 30–40 minute practice and then do between 10 and 20 minutes on the other days that is a great place to start.

KEEPING A JOURNAL

As you begin your fertility yoga journey, we recommend that you begin to keep a journal to keep track of how your practice is going as well as write down goals, affirmations or any emotions or feelings you want to release on paper. Your journal can be used to keep track of your cycle and how it changes with the fertility yoga program and other modalities you might be trying like acupuncture or fertility abdominal massage. You may also decide to make some lifestyle changes like altering your diet, and a journal is a great way to record the changes you are making and how they might be impacting how you feel. Free-form writing can be a wonderful way

Exercise to Help Open the Body-to-Mind Communication Channel During Yoga

In our classes, we encourage students to pay attention to what they are feeling in their bodies as a result of the yoga poses, in order to get practice at body-to-mind communication. Some questions you could ask yourself as you do the routines in this book include:
- Where am I feeling this pose in my body?
- Does the second side of pose feel the same as or different than the first side?
- Am I able to breathe freely and evenly in this pose? (If not, try backing out of the pose a bit and see if that improves the breath.)
- Where is my mind at this moment? (If it is somewhere else, see if you can just invite it back to your yoga mat, without judging yourself.)

to get in touch with yourself and help you to determine in which direction you need to go when faced with challenging decisions. There is no right way to keep a journal, so keep in mind that you can use it in any way that feels right to you.

BASIC YOGA PRINCIPLES

Before you begin, we would like to share some of our basic principles about practicing yoga for you to think about as you are doing the routines. These might be characterized as underlying attitudes that we believe are important to bring to a yoga practice, and that will help you get the most value from your practice.

1. **Work in your comfort zone**. Do what you can do; never force it. Stretch only as far as feels comfortable. The point of the poses is not to do the maximum possible in any given pose. It would be much better to find a place to be in the pose where you can breathe and stay focused. Remember that in yoga the journey is more important than the destination—you might even say that the journey IS the destination.

2. **Accept and respect what you can do without judging**. This principle carries with it three very important principles of yoga: acceptance, respect for yourself, and letting go of judgment. This may be the most difficult principle, because we are so used to doing the opposite.

3. **Don't worry about how you look in the poses**. As we mentioned earlier, the models in the book are very experienced yoga practitioners. Your poses may not look much like theirs in the beginning. However, the form is less important in the poses than the ability to breathe and move energy. Although it may be tempting to practice in front of a mirror, and this may be valuable sometimes, it would be preferable not to do this. We as a culture tend to be very visually and externally oriented. In yoga, we try to cultivate a more internally oriented frame of reference.

4. **Listen to your body**. This is a particularly important skill to practice

when you are trying to conceive. Our body has important messages for us, but we have to be paying attention in order to hear them. As you try the yoga poses, see if you can tune in to the feedback your body is giving you for each pose. Notice where you feel each pose, and which poses feel best to you.

5. **Be present.** In order to listen to your body, you will need to keep your mind and your body in the same place at the same time. This is perhaps the most difficult practice to implement because we rarely do it. Try, as you do the poses, to have your mind present and focused on what you are doing. If you notice your mind wandering—which you will!—simply notice that and bring it back to focus on the pose you are in, and notice any sensation you are feeling in the pose. Let go of any self-judgment. Even very seasoned yogis struggle and find their minds wandering pretty frequently!

As you work with this practice, you will find that it reduces stress and promotes a calm, centered feeling. This is because 98% of our stress comes not from the current moment, but from worries about past or future events. Giving ourselves a break from being drawn into the past and future has big benefits for de-stressing.

6. **Breathe fully and deeply.** Each routine begins with a breathing practice. This is a way to remind the body to take full advantage of the available breathing space in the body, so that, as you go through the poses, your breath will continue to be full and deep. Pay attention to your breath as you are in each pose. The breath is a good clue to

how you are doing in the pose. If you notice you are holding your breath, or unable to take nice, deep inhales and exhales, you may be pushing yourself too far in the pose. Back out of the pose a bit, and see if you can get back to a place where you can take smooth, even breaths.

7. **Rest as you need to.** There is no benefit whatsoever in getting through the routines quickly. Take your time in each pose, and rest between poses if you feel the need to do so. It is also not necessary to do the entire routine. If you are unable to do the whole routine, you can simply choose a few poses to do.

8. **Yoga should feel good!** Come out of the pose if it feels really uncomfortable or painful. You may feel a stretch in a particular set of muscles, and this kind of "discomfort" is fine. But if a pose really feels uncomfortable or painful, it would be better not to do it at this point. Particularly if you have injuries, pay attention to those, and don't do poses that exacerbate them. We need to release our Western idea of "no pain, no gain," because it doesn't apply to fertility yoga.

9. **What you focus on expands.** Pay attention to what you focus on as you practice. If you focus on the discomfort, it will increase. If you focus on the breath, it will expand. This is also a good life principle to practice: be careful what you focus on, because that is what will expand in your life. If you are always focusing on negative things, you will draw more of these kinds of things into your life. If you choose positive things to focus on, that is what you will draw to yourself.

Our Basic Principles of Yoga Practice

- Work in your comfort zone.
- Accept and respect what you can do without judging.
- Pay more attention to the breath than to how you look.
- Listen to your body.
- Be present.
- Breathe fully and deeply.
- Rest as you need to.
- Yoga should feel good!
- What you focus on expands.

Now, you are ready to begin your yoga for fertility practice!

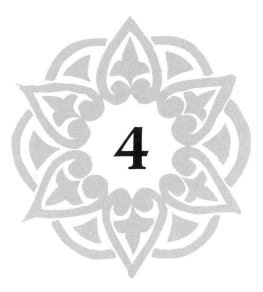

Yoga for Fertility: Routines for the First Half of Your Cycle

YOGA FOR FERTILITY: FIRST HALF BASIC ROUTINE

The following sequence of basic fertility yoga poses are ideally performed from the end of your period to the time of ovulation. *(Once you have ovulated, you can move to the Basic Poses in the Second Half Routine.)* The poses with a double asterisk in this routine should not be performed during the main flow days of your period. There is a yoga routine in Chapter 6 specifically designed to be performed during your period. If you are not sure of the exact timing of ovulation, just use your best judgment. If you really don't know which half of your cycle you are in, we recommend that you use the Second Half Basic Routine in the next chapter, as a more cautious choice. You can refer to Chapter 3 for more information on determining the timing of your cycle and more guidance on deciding which practice is best suited for you.

Before you begin this practice, please read through the "Getting Started" section of Chapter 3, which explains what equipment you will need and provides other important information. The first section of photos, called "Summary Flow", is a quick look at the routine, designed to show how the poses follow each other. After this section, each pose is explained in further detail, including how to set up the pose, and its benefits.

SUMMARY FLOW OF FIRST HALF BASIC ROUTINE

Note: A double asterisk ** means you should not practice this pose during the main flow days of your period.

1. **Centering/Calming Breath (Belly Breath)**

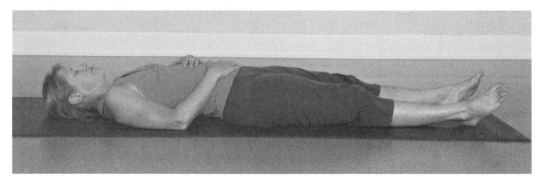

2. **Sacrum Circles**

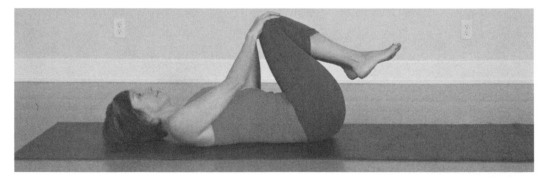

3. **Pelvic Tilts**

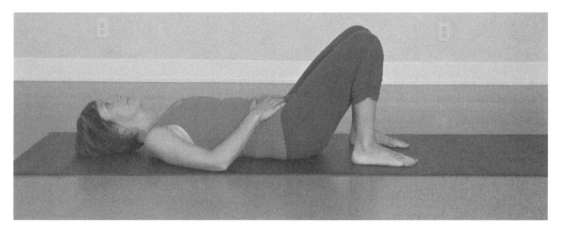

4. **Outer Hip Stretch (#4 pose)**

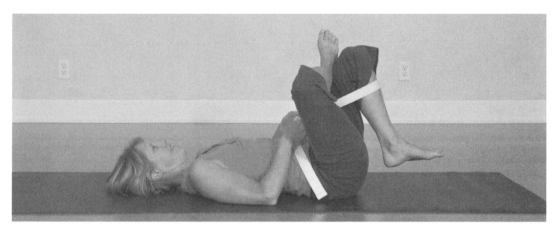

5. **Reclined Cobbler Pose**

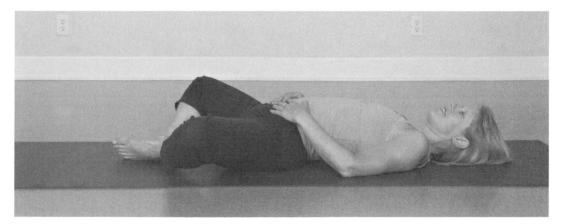

6. Bent Knee Twist (First Half Version)

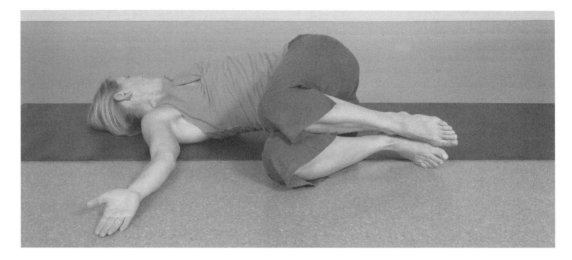

7. Coming Up

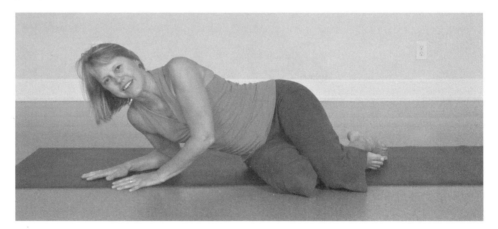

8. Cat-Cow

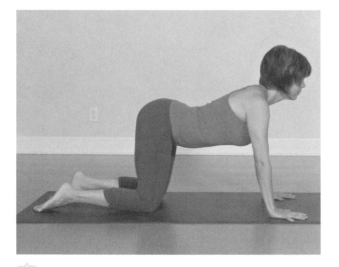 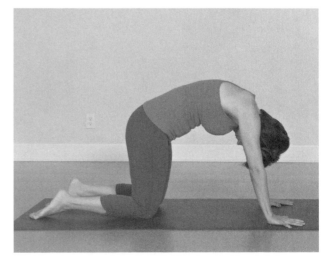

9. **Cat-Cow Circles**

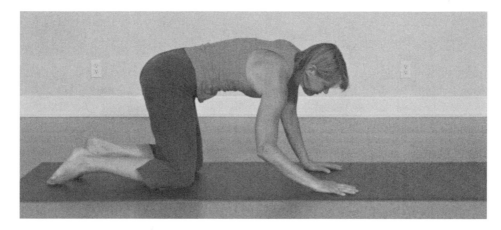

10. **Prayer Pose (Child's Pose)**

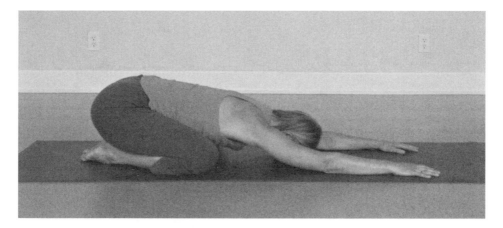

11. **Downward Facing Dog**

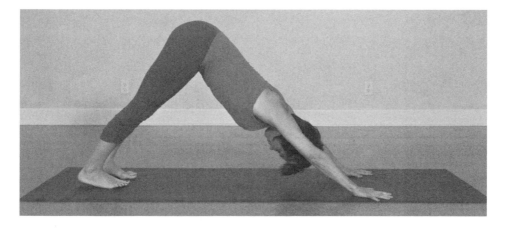

12. **Variation of Prayer Pose (Child's Pose)**

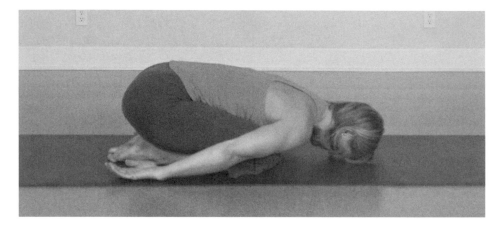

13. ****Moving Cobra**

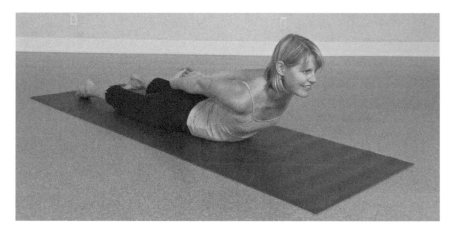

14. ****Moving Sphinx**

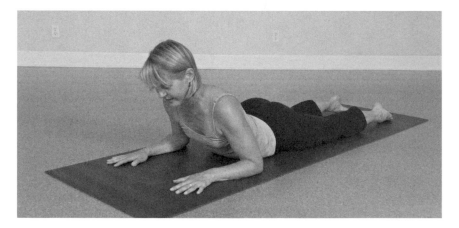

15. ****Locust**

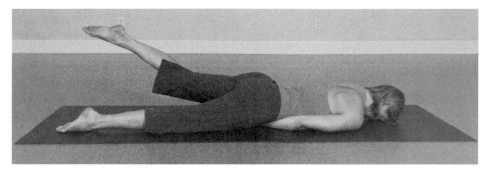

16. **Prayer Pose Variation**

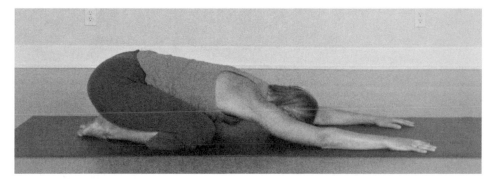

17. **Knee-Down Lunge**

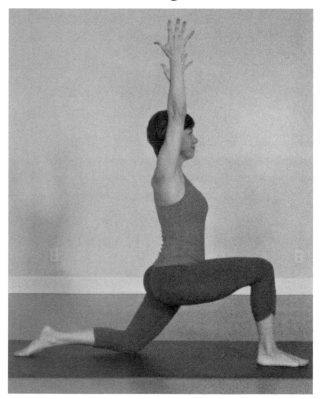

18. **Mountain Pose**

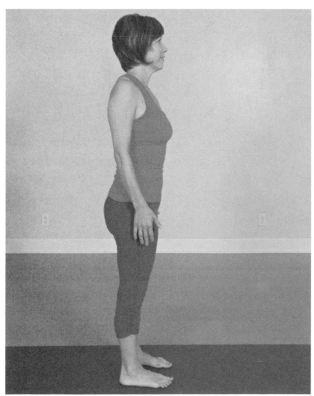

19. Standing Hip Circles

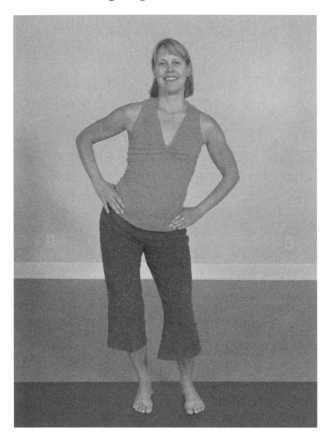

20. Tree Pose

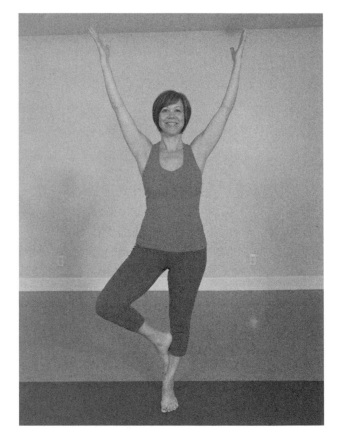

21. Wide Standing Forward Bend

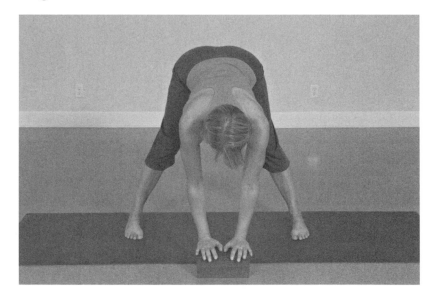

22. Wide Standing Forward Bend with Twist

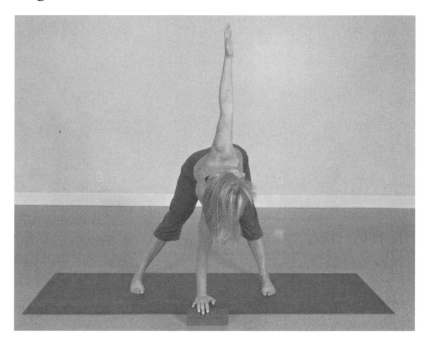

23. Coming Up to Standing

24. "Chicken Wing" Shoulder Stretch

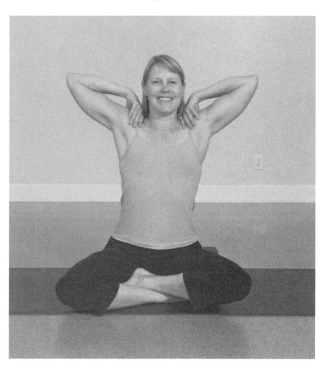

25. Cobbler Pose with Heart Opener

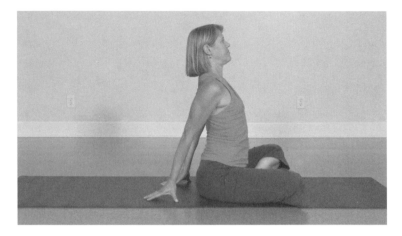

26. **Pelvic Floor Contractions

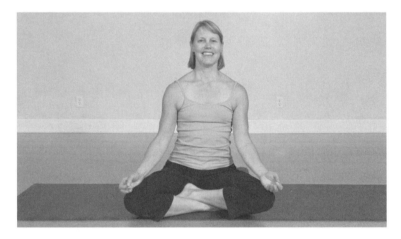

27. Seated Spinal Twist

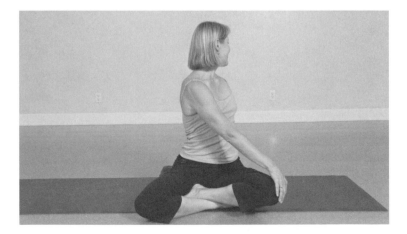

28. **Legs Up the Wall

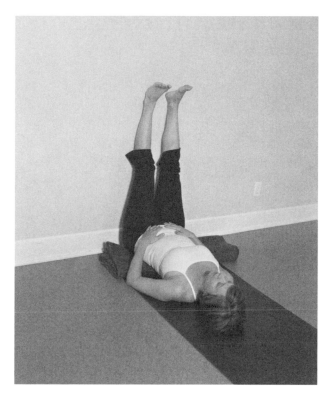

29. Corpse Pose

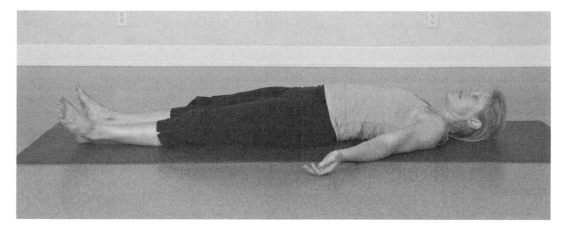

✦ POSE DESCRIPTIONS FOR FIRST HALF BASIC ROUTINE

I. CENTERING/CALMING BREATH (BELLY BREATH)

Setup

This breath can be performed either seated or lying down. Lie down on your back on your mat with your legs straight, or bend the knees if that is more comfortable for the low back. Another option is to sit in a chair with a solid seat that will allow you to sit with a long spine. Let your body relax and place your hands on your low belly.

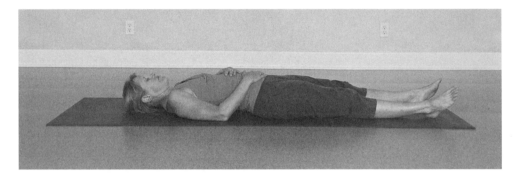

Movement

Breathe fully and deeply into your abdominal region, visualizing the prana (life force energy) filling your belly and creating the loving, open space for life. On the exhalations, visualize stress, defeating thoughts, frustration, etc., all leaving the body. Feel the muscles relax and get heavy with each exhalation. On the inhalations, invite the prana into every cell of your body. Feel your hands rise with your breath. Let the gentle rhythm of your breath take you deeper and deeper into relaxation. Set an intention related to your fertility journey. This can be as simple as "I intend to get pregnant and have a beautiful, healthy baby." It can also be something like, "I intend to be kind to myself in this process of trying to conceive." Continue this breathing until you feel calm, and the breath is smooth and even. Ideally, the inhale and exhale should be either equal in length, or the exhale should be a little longer. Allow there to be a bit of a pause at the end of the exhale, and the end of the inhale, before you start the next breath. This "space" is perhaps the most important part of the breath. Try at least 12 full inhales and exhales, but feel free to do more if your mind hasn't calmed after 12 breaths.

Why Do This?

This centering/calming breathing technique helps the body and mind relax. The deep, conscious breaths send signals to the nervous system that the muscles in the body can relax, and the mind can stop racing. Allowing the breath to expand the low belly helps us overcome cultural conditioning to hold in the abdomen, and helps to release tension in the pelvic area. Deep breathing is a wonderful way to begin your yoga practice. It can also be used on its own as a technique any time you need to relax.

POSES LYING ON YOUR BACK

2. SACRUM CIRCLES

Setup

Lie on your back, bend the knees and take the feet up off the floor.

Movement

Put the hands onto the knees and gently circle the knees one direction, keeping a nice even breath going with the circles. Try to make this mostly about the breath, with the movement just following the lead of the breath. After a few circles, pause and switch directions.

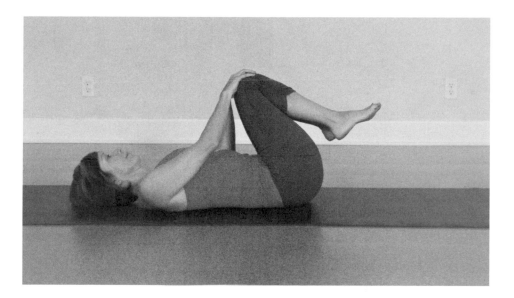

Why Do This?

This action massages the sacrum, which is the flat bone on the low back, at the lower end of the spine. In the yoga "map" of the body, the sacrum is part of the reproductive energy center, so keeping circulation and energy moving through this area is important. It is also a chance to practice adding a simple movement to the breath, while maintaining your focus on the breath.

3. PELVIC TILTS

Setup

While lying on your back, release the feet down to the floor. Your feet should be hip-width apart (4–6 inches) and parallel.

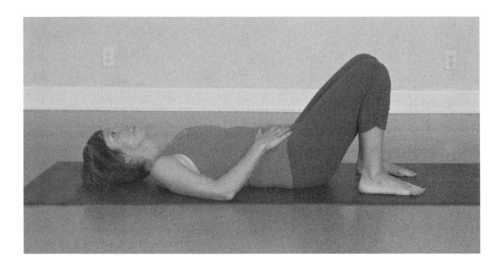

Movement

With an exhale, *gently* tilt the pelvis to press the low back down into the floor. On the inhale release and let the low back come up again. Repeat 5–8 times.

Why Do This?

While there are versions of this pose that are used for core strengthening, that is not our purpose here. We are using this pose to create a gentle rocking of the pelvis. This encourages blood and energy flow, and releases tension and stagnation in the pelvis. For this purpose, press the low back down *gently*, trying not to engage the abdominal muscles any more than necessary to get the action to happen.

4. OUTER HIP STRETCH (#4 POSE)

Setup

Find your strap. With your knees bent and feet on the floor, lift the left foot, and pass the strap around the left shin. Release the right foot back to the floor. Hold one end of the strap in each hand. Now, cross the right ankle inside the left knee. One end of the strap should come through the triangular space in the center between the two legs.

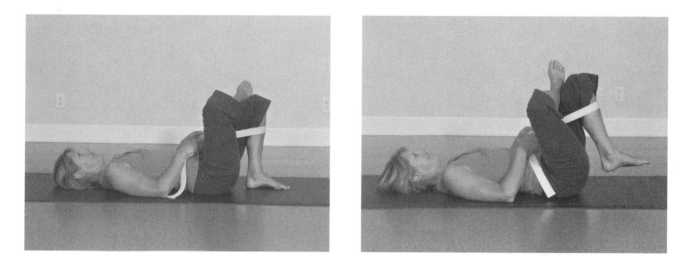

Movement

If you are already feeling a lot of stretch in the right outer hip or hamstring area, just keep the left foot on the floor and breathe. For more stretch, pull on the straps to draw the left knee gently toward the chest. Breathe with full, even breaths. Try 5–8 breaths here. Switch the legs and do the other side of the pose. Let the shoulders relax as much as possible while holding the strap. Relax the face muscles, too. See how many muscles in the body you can relax while allowing the outer hip rotators to stretch. (*Modification:* If you have knee injuries, don't take the strap around the shin. Instead, pass the strap under the knee).

Why Do This?

We are stretching the rotator muscles in the outer hips, which are a group of short, but powerful muscles that are tight on many people. This is because just about everything we do on a regular basis tightens them—including walking, sitting, and many other common, everyday activities. Releasing tension in these muscles also releases tension in the pelvic area, and allows energy and blood flow to move more easily through this area.

5. RECLINED COBBLER POSE

Setup

Lying on your back, bring the soles of the feet together to touch.

Movement

Slowly allow your knees to open apart from each other, releasing down toward the floor. Rest your hands on your low belly, or allow them to gently rest by your sides, palms facing up. Take at least 5 to 8 slow, full breaths. If you feel strain in the inner groin or knees, you can place a pillow or folded blanket under each knee for extra support.

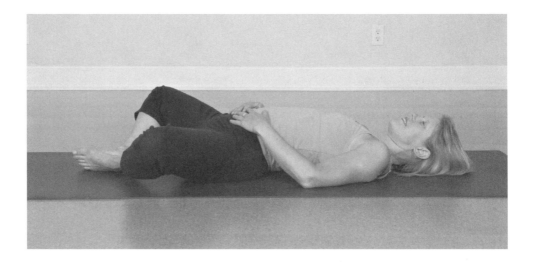

Why Do This?

This pose opens and relaxes the whole pelvic bowl, allowing the organs of the pelvic bowl to release any tension they are holding. It is a great pose to do if you are having any menstrual or uterine cramping. It is also a counter-pose to the outer hip stretch we did in the previous pose.

6. BENT KNEE TWIST (FIRST HALF VERSION)

Setup

With your knees bent and feet on the floor, take the feet to the outer edges of your yoga mat. The feet will be about two feet apart. Now, take the arms out to the sides like a "T," with your palms facing up.

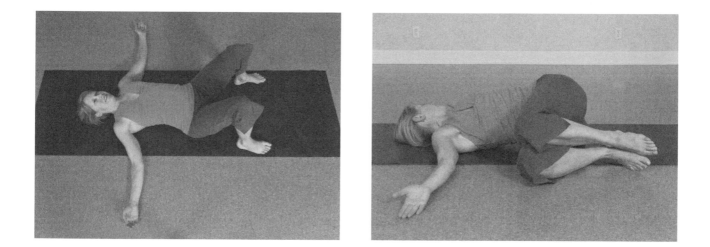

Movement

Lift the hips and shift them slightly toward the left. Then allow the knees to drop slowly over toward the right. Pick up the left knee and place it on top of the right knee. The knees can come all the way to the floor, if your ribcage and back allow. You may find a trade-off between the knees coming to the floor, and the opposite shoulder coming off the ground. In this case, allow the knees to come down, and then try to release the shoulder toward the floor, as you can. Turn the head to look back toward the left palm. Take several slow, even breaths. On an inhale, bring the knees back to center, and do the twist to the second side.

Why Do This?

Twists like this are cleansing and rejuvenating for the organs (such as the uterus and intestines) and glands (such as the ovaries) in the abdominal area. Basically, as you twist, the blood is squeezed out of those organs and glands like wringing out a sponge. As you come out of the twist, a fresh blood supply is delivered to them, nourishing the organs and glands.

7. COMING UP

Setup

To prepare for the next set of poses, bend your knees and roll onto your right side. Take a breath or two on your right side.

Movement

Use both hands to gently press yourself back up to a seated position.

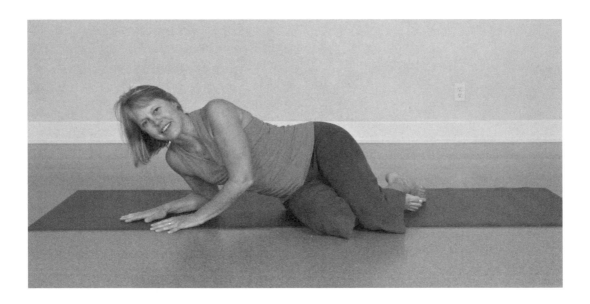

Why Do This?

Rolling to the side and pressing the floor inhibits tension in the neck and lower back. Rolling to the right side keeps the heart on top, so that you don't compress the heart (which is located on the left side). It also keeps the pulse regular, and frees up the breath through the left nostril, which promotes relaxation.

POSES ON HANDS AND KNEES

8. CAT-COW

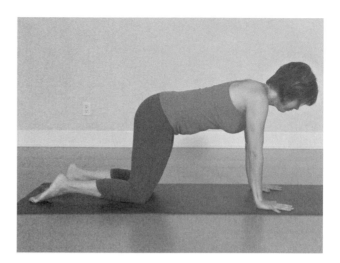

Setup

Come onto your hands and knees with your wrists underneath your shoulders and your knees underneath your hips. Spread the fingers wide apart from each other. Your knees should be about 4–6 inches apart. If this position bothers your knees, you can try folding a blanket and placing it underneath your knees for extra padding.

Movement

On an inhale, tilt your tailbone up and arch your back. Look forward and draw the shoulders back away from the ears. Keep your core engaged as you arch the back. On an exhale, tilt your tailbone down toward the floor and round your spine. Press the shoulder blades up toward the ceiling. Let your head and neck feel heavy. Repeat at least 5 times, initiating each movement at the tailbone. Allow the movement to follow the breath.

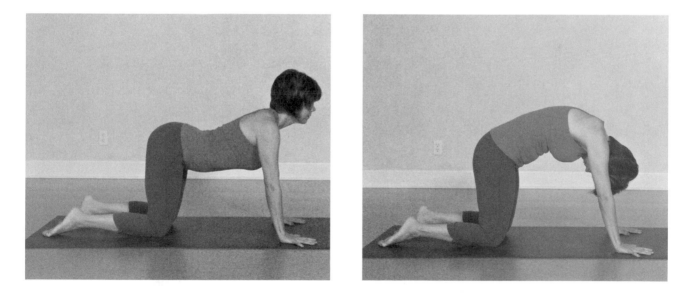

Why Do This?

Cat-cow warms up all of the muscles in the back and allows tension in the neck and shoulders to release. It also opens the major energy channels in the front and back of the body. The pelvic movements bring blood flow and energy through the pelvis.

9. CAT-COW CIRCLES

Setup

Setup is the same as for Cat-Cow.

Movement

Circle the hips and ribcage around to the right, bending the elbows as much as you need to. This is a very free-form movement, so just do what feels good to your body. You may get some forward-and-back movement as well as the circling. Don't forget to breathe while performing these circles. After a few breaths, switch directions.

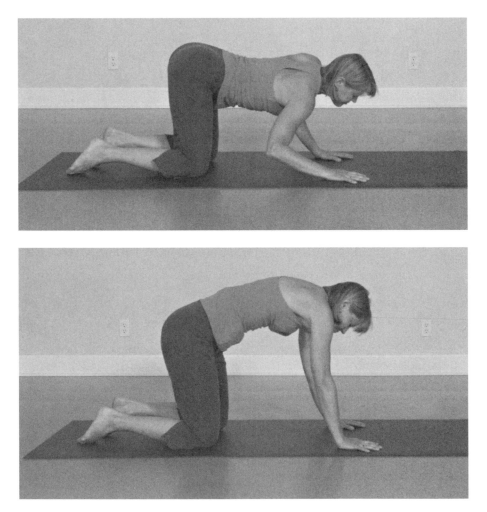

Why Do This?

The circling motion releases tension in the pelvis, ribcage and shoulders. We are taking the torso through a range of motion that most of us don't experience in our regular daily lives, so it encourages us to release physical and emotional patterns where we may be "stuck."

10. PRAYER POSE (CHILD'S POSE)

Setup

From the hands and knees position, take the knees wide apart and sit the hips back onto the heels. Keep the toes together. Bring the forehead to the floor, and reach the arms forward with the palms facing down. If it isn't comfortable to bring the forehead all the way to the floor, you can stack the hands one on top of the other, and rest the forehead on the hands, or rest the forehead on a block or a folded blanket. Let the toes release.

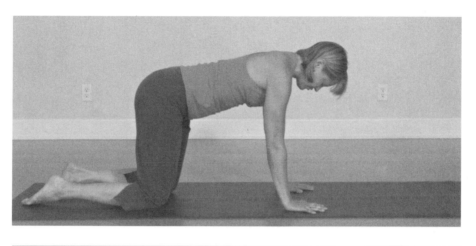

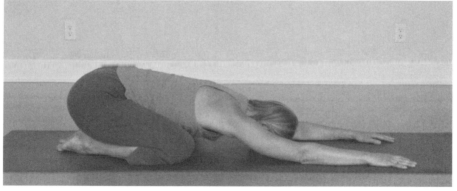

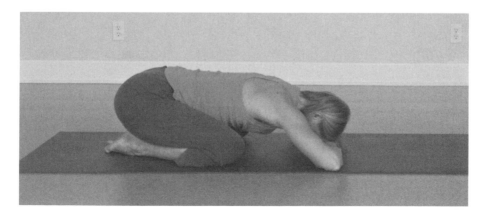

Movement

Prayer pose is a resting pose, so in the standard version of prayer pose, you are resting here, rather than moving. To come up from prayer pose, just walk the hands back in toward the body, and come up slowly.

Variations

Try a couple of variations of prayer pose that include some movement: *Variation 1)* In prayer pose, gently and slowly move the hips side to side, stretching out each side of the low back. *Variation 2)* On an exhale, creep the hands over to the right side of the mat, or even past the mat, until you get a stretch in the left side of the body. You can optionally turn the head and look toward the right, to get some stretch into the neck. Take a few breaths here. On an inhale, creep the hands back to center, and on the next exhale, repeat the pose on the left side.

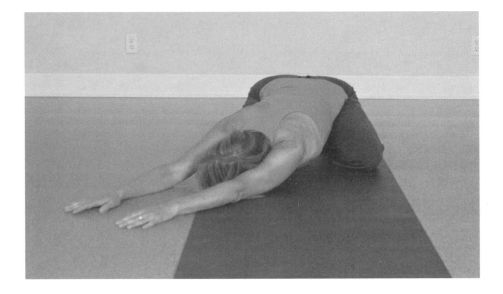

Why Do This?

Prayer pose is known for its calming effect, which is due to resting the forehead down. It also stretches and relaxes the low back and opens the shoulders.

11. DOWNWARD FACING DOG

Setup

From the hands and knees position, take an inhale and engage the muscles of the arms. Relax the space between your shoulder blades.

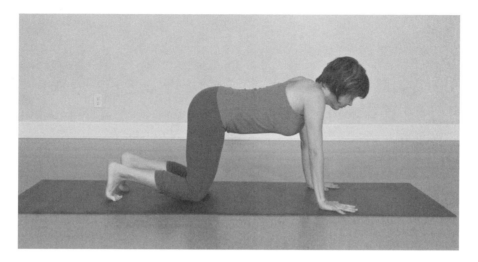

Movement

Exhale, curl your toes under and lift your knees off of the floor. Lift the hips, and draw the low belly up and back. Press strongly through the hands, and draw energy from the hands up the arms. Take a peek back at your feet and be sure they are "sitting-bones-width" distance apart (about 4–6 inches apart) and parallel. Keep the undersides of the arms lifting away from the floor. Your heels may or may not touch the floor. If you feel a lot of stretch in your hamstrings, bend the knees slightly, allowing the back to lengthen. Stay here for 3 to 5 breaths feeling the whole body stretch and lengthen. Then inhale, bend the knees, and return to the hands and knees position. **Don't do this pose if you are on your period.**

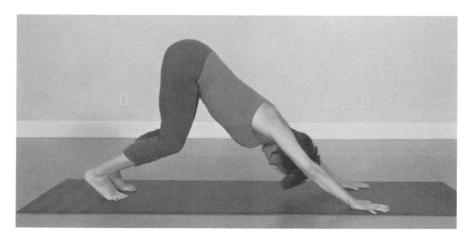

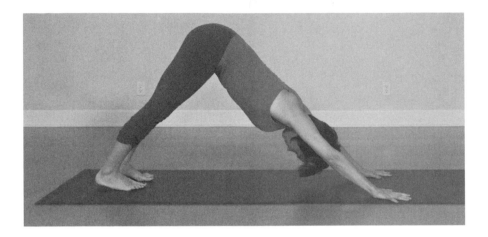

Why Do This?

Downward facing dog is a full body stretch that is good for the whole body. It is also a partial inversion, which is beneficial for the circulatory system as well as for the endocrine system. It tones the abdominal muscles, opens the shoulders, and can help regulate problems with the menstrual cycle. However, you should not do this pose for an extended period of time during the main flow days of your period. From a fertility perspective, it opens the energy channel between the heart and the uterus. In the Chinese medicine tradition, opening this energy channel is one of the keys to conception.

12. VARIATION OF PRAYER POSE (CHILD'S POSE)

Setup

Setup is the same as for prayer pose, except that the arms reach back along the outside of the calves, rather than reaching forward. The benefits are similar to those of prayer pose.

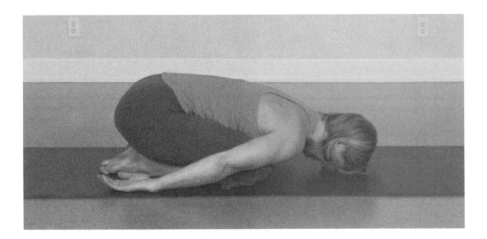

✤ SUPINE POSES AND LUNGE POSE

13. **MOVING COBRA

Setup

Lie on your belly with the forehead resting on the floor. Clasp your hands behind your back.

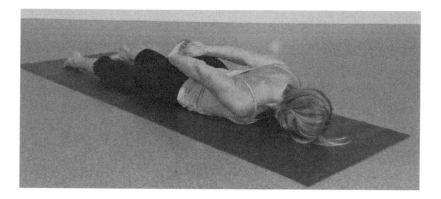

Movement

On an inhale, raise the head and shoulders up away from the floor. Keep the eyes looking down at the floor, to keep the back of the neck long. Exhale, and lower your head and shoulders back down on the floor. Repeat 4–6 times. **Don't do this pose if you are on your period**.

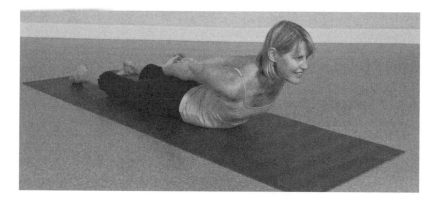

Why Do This?

This pose is very stimulating, cleansing and nourishing for the ovaries and abdominal organs. When you rise up, you compress the belly and squeeze the blood out of the organs. As you lower the body back down, the organs receive a fresh blood supply.

14. **MOVING SPHINX

Setup

Lying on your belly, rest the forehead on the floor. Allow the forearms and hands to rest on the floor, with the elbows in near the body.

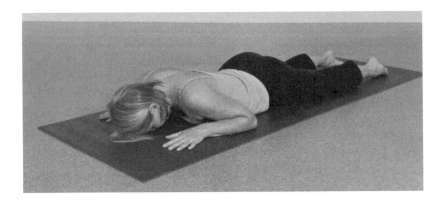

Movement

On an inhale, press through the hands and forearms, and raise the head and shoulders up away from the floor. Keep the eyes looking down at the floor, to keep the back of the neck long. Exhale, and lower back down. Repeat 4–6 times. **Don't do this pose if you are on your period**.

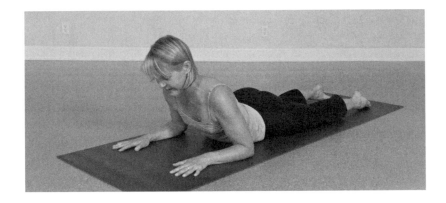

Why Do This?

The benefits of this pose are similar to those of the Moving Cobra.

15. **LOCUST

Setup

Lie on your belly with the forehead resting on the floor. Make your hands into fists and tuck them underneath your body, palms facing up. Place them so that the middle joints of the fingers touch the pubic bone, and the thumbs touch each other. Make sure the forearms are to the inside of the hip bones (ASIS bones), and not underneath the bones, or this will be very uncomfortable.

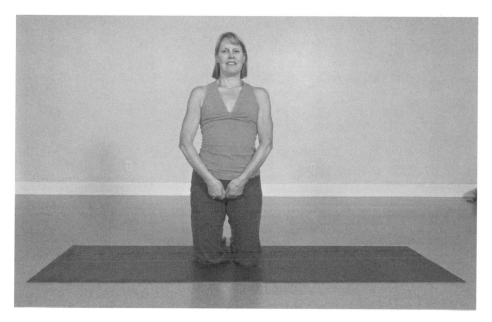

Movement

On the inhale, raise the right leg up away from the floor. Be careful not to raise the hip or tilt the pelvis—just raise the leg, without bending the knee. Keep the forehead resting on the mat. Exhale, and lower the leg. Continue, alternating between the right and left leg. Do a total of 4 lifts for each leg. **Don't do this pose if you are in the main flow days of your period**. *More advanced:* Try raising both legs together and holding them up for 3 breaths. Then lower the legs and rest.

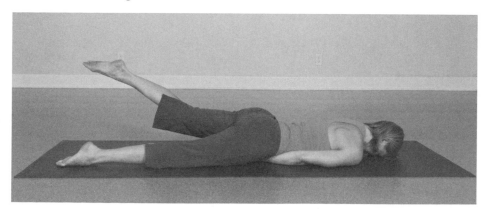

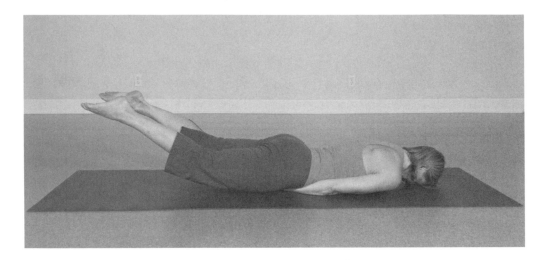

Why Do This?

This pose is very stimulating for the ovaries and abdominal organs. When you raise the leg, the fists compress the area of the low belly containing the ovaries and uterus. This stimulates circulation and energy flow, and as you lower the leg, the organs receive a fresh blood supply.

16. PRAYER POSE (CHILD'S POSE)

Setup

Setup is the same as for Prayer Pose. Move hips gently side-to-side in prayer pose to release low back.

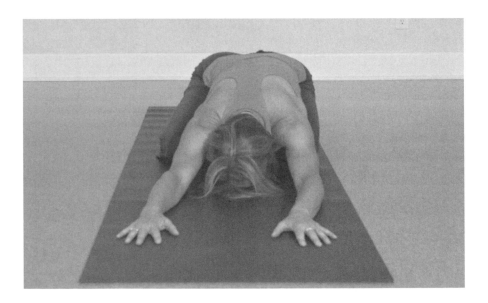

17. KNEE-DOWN LUNGE

Setup

From prayer pose, walk your hands back in toward your body, raising your torso.

Movement

Step your right foot forward between your hands and curl your back toes under so you are pressing the ball of the left foot into the floor. Squeeze the legs in toward an imaginary midline down the center of your body. The hands can remain on the floor, on either side of the front foot, or you can place both hands on your right thigh. Stay here or reach your arms over your head. Take 5 full breaths in this pose. Retrace your steps carefully until you are back to a tabletop position on your hands and knees. Repeat steps on the left side. After the second side, step the right foot forward and come up to a standing position at the front of your mat.

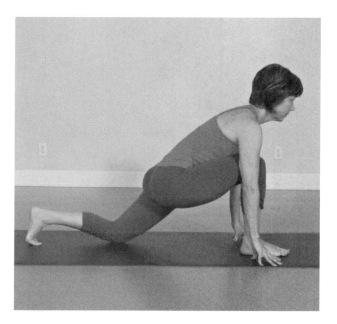

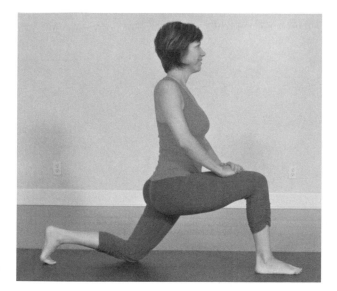

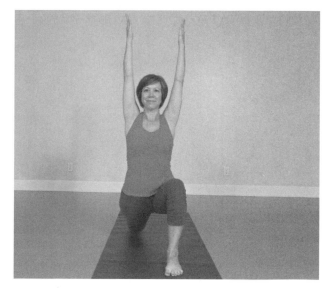

Why Do This?

This pose tones the abdominal organs including the reproductive organs. It opens the quadriceps, which allows more circulation and energy to flow into the pelvic area.

✹ STANDING POSES

18. MOUNTAIN POSE

Setup

Stand with your feet hip-width apart (about 4–6 inches) and parallel. Allow the arms to rest gently by your sides.

Movement

Make sure your feet are not turned out or in. Try to balance the weight evenly on the front and backs of the feet and on the inner and outer edges of the feet. Notice if your knees are collapsing in toward each other and bring the knees over the ankles. Also be sure not to hyperextend your knee joints. Ideally your pelvis will be in a neutral position. Be sure that your shoulders are over your hips and your neck and chin are not jutting out. Lengthen the crown of your head toward the sky and take 5 to 8 breaths.

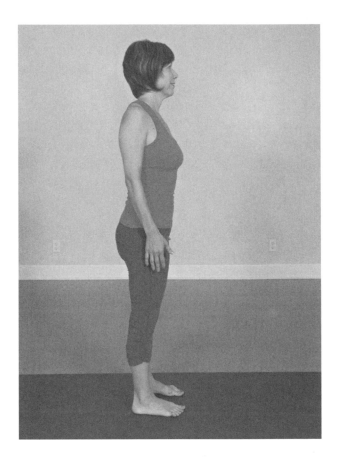

Why Do This?

Mountain pose can be practiced anywhere. It helps you develop body awareness and good posture for breathing. It also tones the abdominal organs.

19. STANDING HIP CIRCLES

Setup

Begin by standing in Mountain Pose.

Movement

Take your hands on your hips, and begin to circle your hips in one direction, bending the knees slightly as you circle. The object of this pose is to get as much range of motion in the hips as you can. Do about 8 circles each direction. Keep a smooth even breath going as you move. Notice if the circles feel easier in one direction than the other.

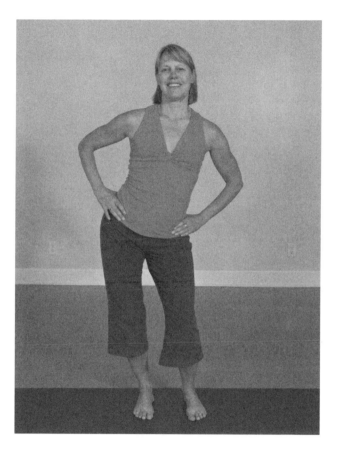

Why Do This?

Hip circles take the hips through a greater range of motion than we get in normal daily activities, which brings more blood flow and energy into the pelvis. These are beneficial for all the pelvic organs.

20. TREE POSE

Setup

Begin by standing in Mountain Pose.

Movement

Bring the weight into your left foot and leg and bend your right knee and place it on your left ankle, calf or thigh. Be careful not to place the foot on the knee joint itself. Bring your palms together in front of your heart. Choose a focal point directly in front of you or on the floor ahead of you. Stay here for 5 to 8 breaths or extend your arms over your head in a V shape and breathe. Retrace your steps slowly to release the pose and repeat on the opposite side.

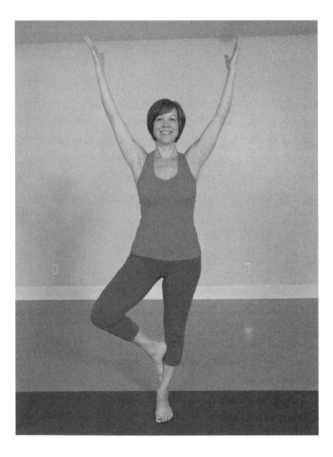 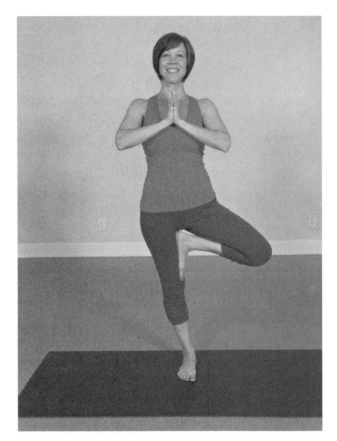

Why Do This?

This pose opens the hips and develops balance, focus, strength and patience. It is a great pose in which to work on the concept of being present during your yoga practice. If your mind wanders in this pose, you usually get instant feedback!

21. WIDE STANDING FORWARD BEND

Setup

Stand with your feet about 3 feet apart, facing one of the long edges of your mat. Place a block in front of you on the floor. Take your hands on your hips. Make sure your feet are parallel to each other.

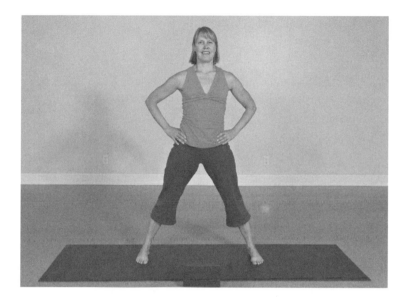

Movement

On an exhale, lean the torso forward from the hip joints. You can bend the knees slightly if your low back feels any strain as you come forward. Release your hands onto the block, which should be placed directly below your shoulders. The arms should be straight, and

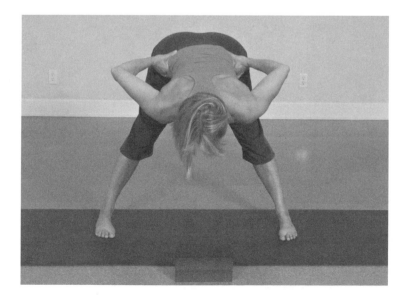

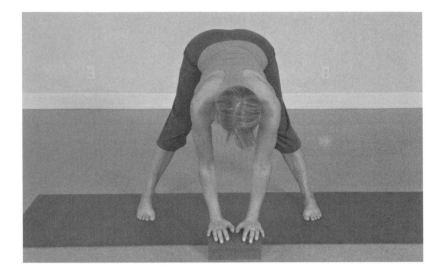

the spine long with the sitting bones reaching back behind you. Adjust the block height if you either can't straighten the arms, or can't keep the spine lengthening. Keep looking toward the floor in order to keep the back of the neck long. The neck should feel like an extension of the rest of the spine. Take 5 to 8 breaths here.

22. WIDE STANDING FORWARD BEND WITH TWIST

Movement

Keep your right hand on the block while you inhale and raise the left arm up toward the ceiling. Turn the head to look toward the left, and allow the torso to open toward the left. Take a few breaths in the pose, then release your hand back down to the block. Perform the twist with the left hand down on the block, opening to the right side.

Why Do This?

This is a great combination pose. The forward bend stimulates the endocrine system while calming the central nervous system. The twist nourishes and stimulates the organs and glands in the abdominal area, including the ovaries and uterus.

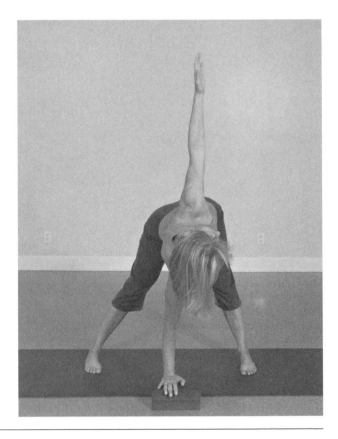

23. COMING UP TO STANDING

Setup

Walk the feet toward each other until they are 6 inches or so apart.

Movement

Bend the knees slightly, let the head and arms hang, and slowly roll up to standing like a rag doll. Try to come up one vertebra at a time. The chin should stay tucked to the chest until you are all the way back to vertical; bring the head up last. If you feel any pain in your low back, place your hands on your hips and come up to standing with a flat back instead.

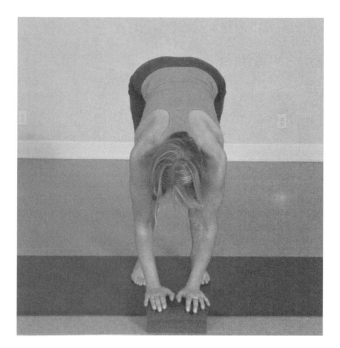

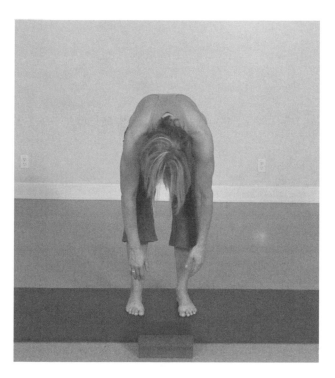

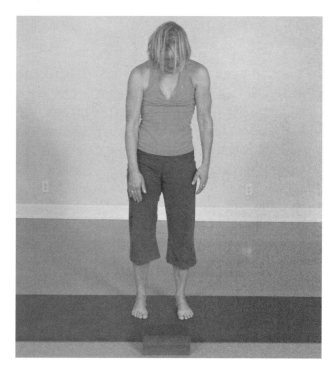

Why Do This?

Rolling up to standing reduces dizziness, as you come up slowly from the forward bend. It also promotes flexibility in the spine.

❋ SEATED POSES

24. "CHICKEN WING" SHOULDER STRETCH

Setup

Come into a comfortable seated, cross-legged position. You may want to sit up on one or two folded blankets if your hips, knees or low back are uncomfortable when sitting on the mat without support. Make sure you are sitting straight down on your sitting bones, not leaning forward or rounding the low back. Take your hands onto your shoulders with the fingers forward, thumbs behind, elbows out to the sides.

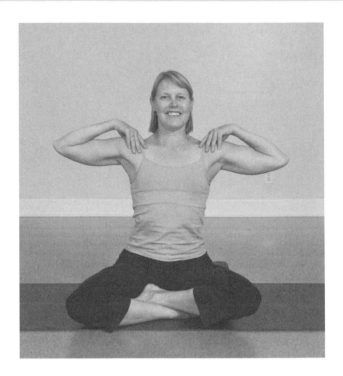

Movement

Inhale and raise the elbows up toward the ceiling. Shrug the shoulders slightly and lengthen the sides of the body. Exhale audibly, through the mouth, lowering the elbows all the way back down next to your rib cage. Repeat 4–6 times.

Why Do This?

This pose reduces shoulder tension, and opens and lengthens the sides of the body, improving blood and energy flow. Audible exhales with the mouth open help clear energy blockages in the throat center, which also helps release pelvic tension.

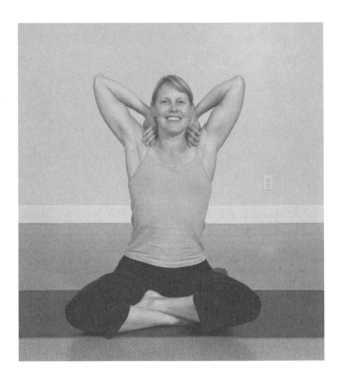

25. COBBLER POSE WITH HEART OPENER

Setup

From your seated position, take the soles of the feet together, gently allowing the knees to open toward the floor.

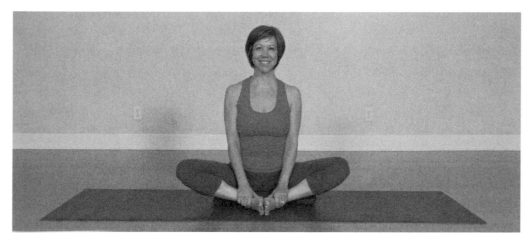

Movement

Place your hands behind your hips on the floor in back of you. On an inhale, lengthen your spine and expand your chest while allowing the knees to open gently down toward the floor. On an exhale, roll your shoulders down and back, and open the heart up toward the ceiling. Stay in the pose for 6–8 breaths.

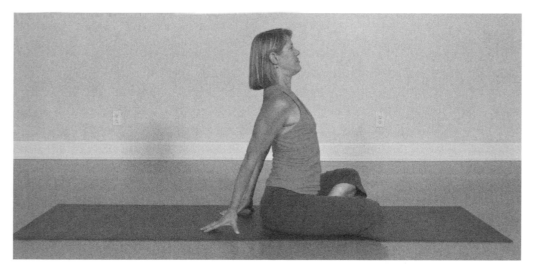

Why Do This?

This pose relaxes the pelvic area, and improves energy flow and blood circulation in the pelvis and heart center. It releases tension in the upper back and shoulders.

26. **PELVIC FLOOR CONTRACTIONS

Setup

Sit on your mat or on a folded blanket in a comfortable, cross-legged position, as for the Chicken Wing Pose. Rest your hands on your knees, and close your eyes. Closing the eyes helps you take your focus internally, rather than externally.

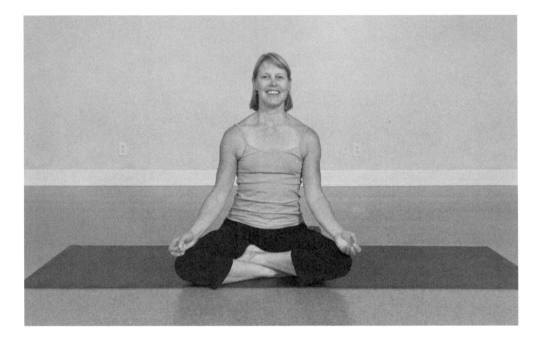

Movement

On an exhale, gently lift the pelvic floor (pubococcygeal, or PC, muscle). The general idea is to *gently* lift and close all the openings in the pelvic floor. On a scale of 1 to 10, with 10 being the hardest you could squeeze the muscles, do this squeeze at about a "6" or a "7". You could imagine trying to pick up a small item with the vaginal opening as you do this. This will help activate all the muscle fibers, which run side-to-side as well as front-to-back. On an inhale, gently release the squeeze, relaxing the pelvic floor as completely as you can. Try this 10 times.

Some Tips:

1. If you want to see if you are doing the correct movement, next time you are in the bathroom, try to stop the flow of urine. When you do that, you are using the same muscles you need to use for the pelvic floor contractions. Just try this once or twice, though—don't practice this pose while urinating.
2. Although it may seem counter-intuitive to lift while exhaling, it actually is easier from a physiological standpoint. The reason is that your diaphragm lifts on exhales, and

drops on inhales. So, if you are lifting the pelvic floor on an exhale, you are going with the prevailing motion of the muscles.

3. If you find it is hard to do 10 of these in a row, or you find your muscles releasing before you inhale, don't worry. The PC muscle is just a muscle like any other in the body—if you haven't been using it in this way, it will be weak. The good news is that our students have reported that in doing this every day for just 2 weeks, they notice it strengthening rather quickly. ****Don't do this pose if you are on the flow days of your monthly period, or if you are constipated**.

Why Do This?

There are many reasons to do pelvic floor exercises. From a fertility standpoint, pelvic floor contractions bring additional blood flow to the pelvic area, which improves the health of the pelvic organs. This is especially useful if we are in jobs where we sit a lot during the day. Since our goal is pregnancy, it makes sense to begin strengthening the pelvic floor now—before we start adding weight down on it. Doing these exercises will help support the extra weight during pregnancy, and provide extra core strength for the birth process. Many women learn these after the birth, to restore the pelvic floor tone; however, it is much easier to restore tone to a muscle that is already toned to begin with.

Pelvic floor exercises are also the best way to prevent stress incontinence, which affects a very high percentage of women following birth, and also following menopause. Pelvic floor exercises also improve sexual function in both women and men. They need not be confined to your yoga routine. You can do these anywhere, anytime. I recommend that my students use those otherwise unproductive minutes when you are standing in line at the grocery store, or waiting for a red light, or sitting in a meeting, to strengthen this important part of the pelvis.

27. SEATED SPINAL TWIST

Setup

Remain sitting on your mat in a comfortable, cross-legged position. As you do the twist, be aware of keeping the spine straight and long.

Movement

On an inhale, reach down through the sitting bones, and up through the crown of the head. Take your left hand onto your right knee, and place your right hand behind you on the floor or on the blanket if you are sitting on one. The hand placement should be just a few inches behind you—not so far behind that you need to lean back to put the hand down. On the exhale, begin to twist to the right. Try turning first with the belly, then the shoulder, and finally following with the head, keeping the movement smooth. Keep the chin level as you turn. On your next inhale, back out of the twist slightly, and with the exhale twist again. Try to keep both sitting bones reaching down as you turn. Reverse the hands and twist to the second side.

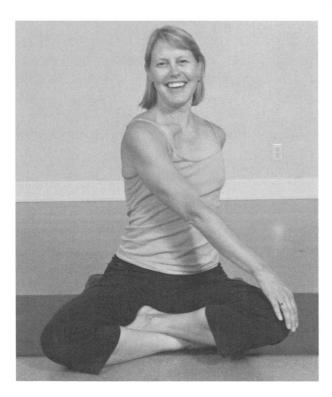 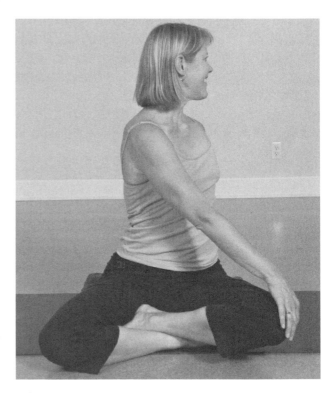

Why Do This?

This twist massages and stimulates the abdominal organs, including the uterus and ovaries. It also balances energy in the body, reduces stress, and relieves tension in the low back, neck and mid-back.

RELAXATION POSES

28. **LEGS UP THE WALL POSE (WITH VARIATIONS)

Setup

Do this pose at a clear space of wall, where you have room to take your legs straight up the wall without bumping into anything. Before you start, put on warm clothes and socks, and have a blanket handy which you can pull over yourself once you get into the pose. Place your yoga mat lengthwise to the wall. Option: place a folded blanket on your mat next to the wall. This can be helpful if your hamstrings are tight or if your low back is uncomfortable in the pose. **Don't do this pose if you are on the main flow days of your period**.

Movement

Start by sitting sideways at the wall, with your right hip just next to the wall and your knees bent. Place your left hand on the floor next to your left hip, and your right hand on the floor behind you. Lean back, and take some weight onto your hands. You might even come down onto your elbows. Next, you will need to swing your legs up the wall, so that your sitting bones end up fairly close to the wall. The actual "best" distance from the wall depends partly on your hamstring flexibility. Find a place where your hamstrings are not unhappy when your legs are up the wall. (If your hamstrings are tight, it may help to place a folded blanket on the mat next to the wall, and sit on the blanket to start. Or, take the sitting bones a little further from the wall.)

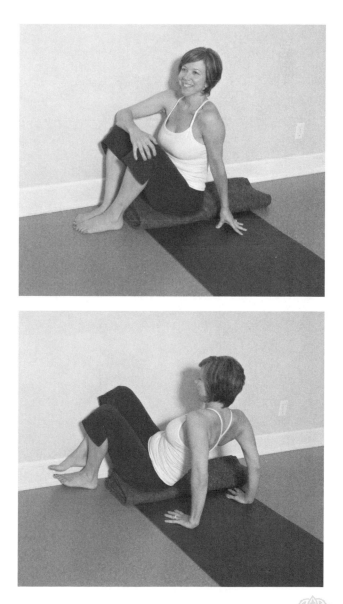

Variations

You can keep the legs a few inches apart on the wall, or try varying the leg position by taking them wider apart, or taking the soles of the feet together like Cobbler Pose. The hands can rest on the low belly, or on either side of you about 12 inches away from the body, with the palms facing up toward the ceiling.

This is a resting pose, so make yourself as comfortable as possible. Take care not to get chilled as you are resting. This pose may take a few practice tries, and may feel awkward at first. This is a very important fertility pose—so don't give up. We recommend you stay in this pose for at least 5 minutes, if you can. When you get ready to come out of the pose, draw the knees into the chest and roll onto your right side with your knees bent. Rest for a few breaths before using both hands to press up to a seated position.

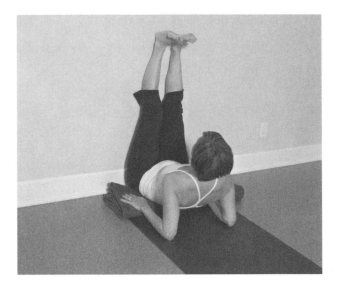

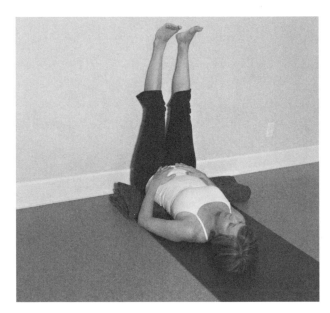

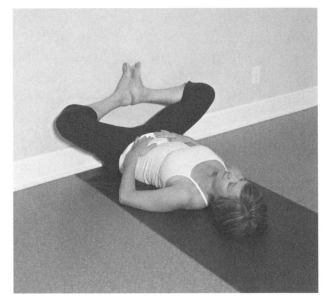

Why Do This?

You may feel like you are doing nothing once you get into the pose, but don't be fooled. This pose is one of the most powerful fertility-supporting yoga poses that you can practice. The abdominal organs are nourished and revitalized when the blood from the feet and legs pools in the low belly. Toxins are removed from the bloodstream, as the blood flows into the lymph glands in the groin. The central nervous system is calmed and the endocrine system is regulated. It is a great pose to do just before bedtime, as it promotes restful sleep. This pose can be done during every part of the cycle except when you are menstruating. However, it is a useful pose if you are trying to get your period to start, or if you are not having regular periods. You may want to choose one of the visualizations from Chapter 7 to do while you are in this pose.

29. CORPSE POSE

Setup

Lie down on your back with your feet and legs relaxed and apart. Allow your arms to rest by your sides a few inches away from your body with your palms facing up. If you have tension or pain in your lower back, place a rolled up blanket or bolster underneath your knees. It is important to stay warm in this pose, so you may want a blanket over you, socks on, etc. For added relaxation, place an eye pillow over your eyes.

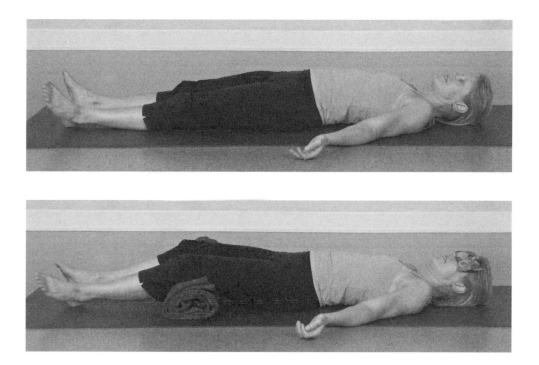

Movement

Feel the support of the floor beneath you, and with each exhale allow your body to feel heavy and relaxed. There is no effort needed here. Tuck your chin ever so slightly toward your chest so the back of the neck is long. Allow your body to rest back into the mat as you relax and open your palms toward the sky, ready to receive the gifts of your practice. If your mind begins to wander, acknowledge that tendency and let the thoughts come and go with each breath. Stay in this pose for 5–7 minutes or even longer if you have time.

Why Do This?

Corpse pose allows all of the benefits of your practice to integrate into your body, mind and spirit. It can help relieve stress and mild depression, and lower blood pressure. Corpse pose can help with insomnia, fatigue and headaches. It also encourages the mind to rest, as the body sinks into a state of deep relaxation.

✿ YOGA FOR FERTILITY: FIRST HALF INTERMEDIATE ROUTINE

The following sequence can be done if you are a more experienced yoga practitioner, or if you have built up your confidence with the Basic Routine.

SUMMARY FLOW OF FIRST HALF INTERMEDIATE ROUTINE

Important Note: A double asterisk (**) means you should not practice this pose during the main flow days of your period.

1. **Centering/Calming Breath (Belly Breath)**

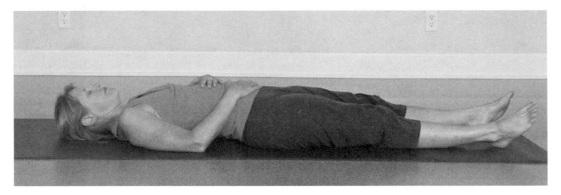

2. **Knees to Chest**

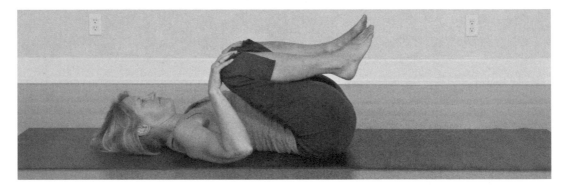

3. **Coming Up**

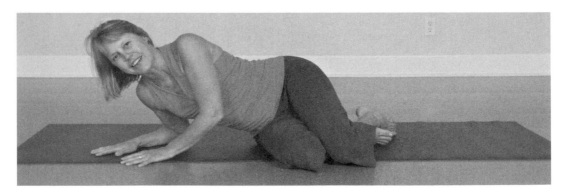

4. Cat-Cow

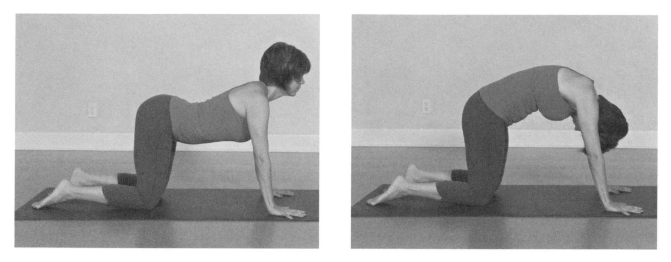

5. Cat-Cow Circles

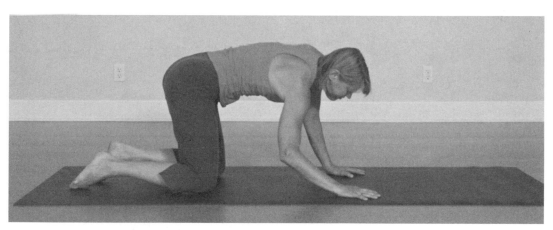

6. **Downward Facing Dog

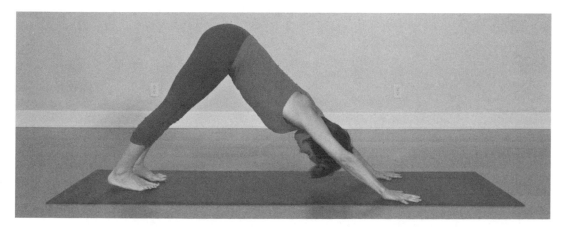

7. **Prayer Pose**

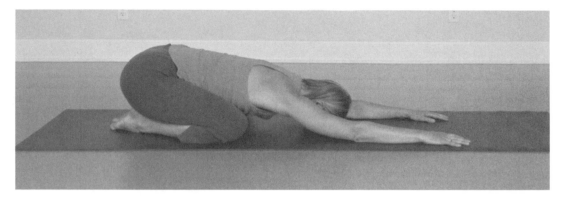

8. **Variation of Prayer Pose (Child's Pose)**

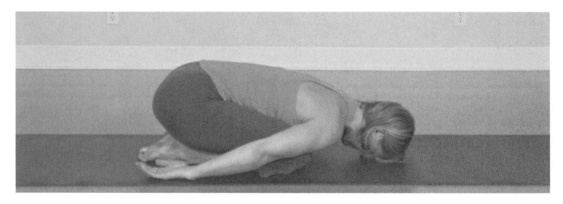

9. **Knee-Down Lunge**

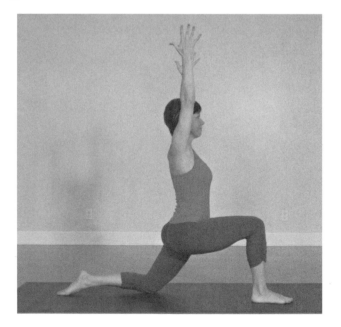

10. Groin Stretch (Lizard Lunge)

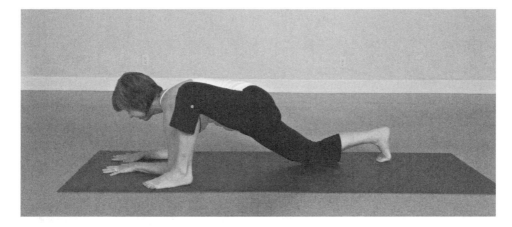

11. Pigeon Pose

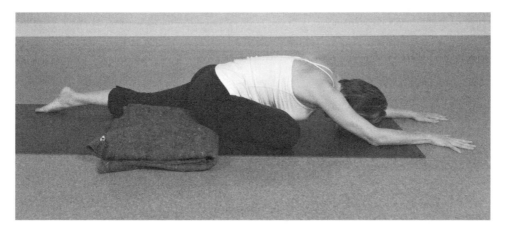

12. *Variation:* Twist in Pigeon Pose

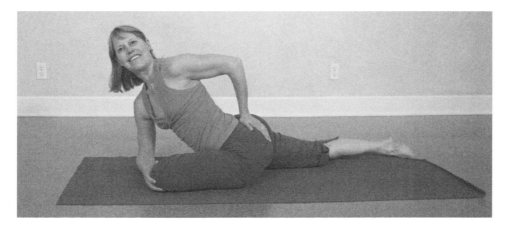

13. **Warrior 2 Pose with Eagle Arms**

14. **Side Angle Pose**

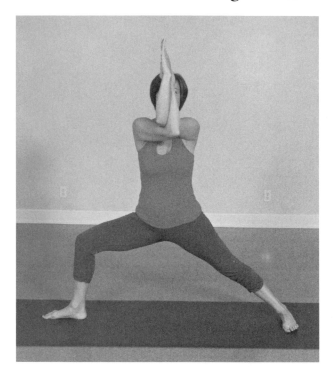

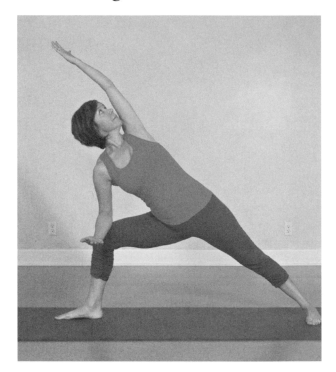

15. **Triangle Pose**

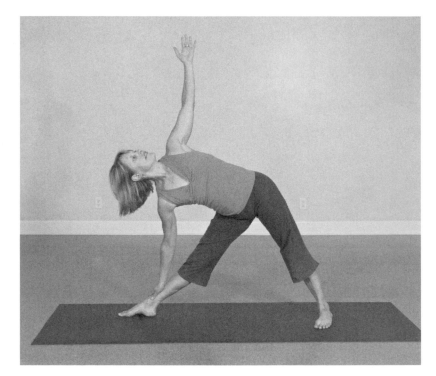

16. **Half-Moon Balance Pose**

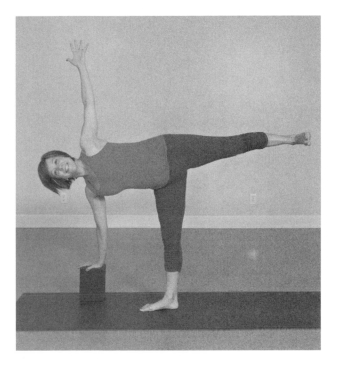

17. **Wide Standing Forward Bend with Immune Booster**

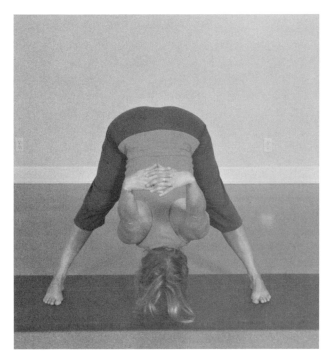

18. ****Moving Cobra**

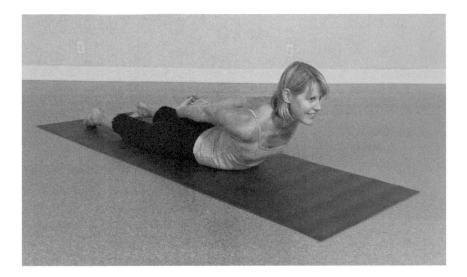

19. **Bow Pose

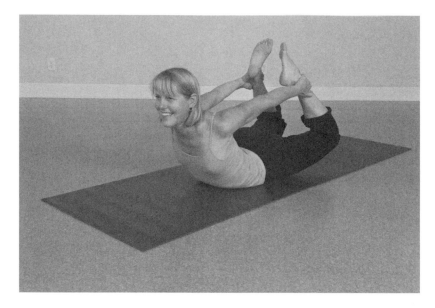

20. **Locust

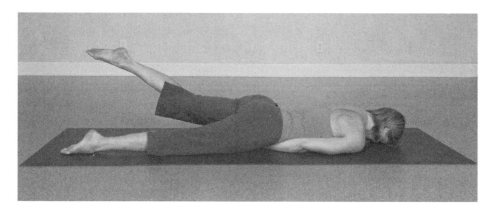

21. Prayer Pose Variation

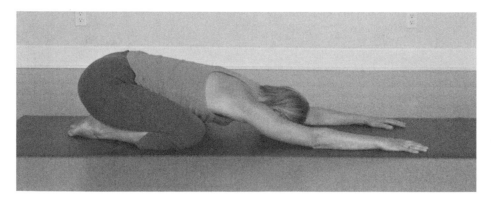

22. **Pelvic Tilts with Floor Contractions

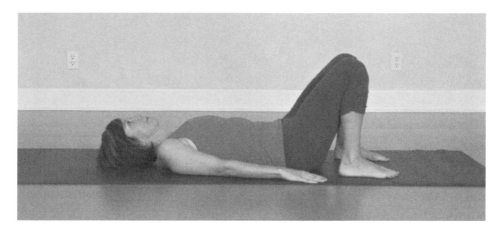

23. **Bridge Pose

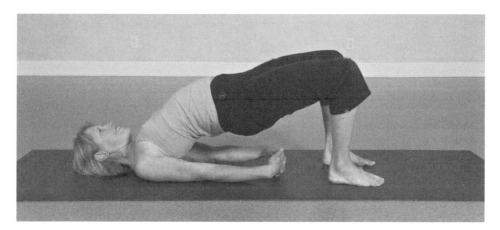

24. Fish Pose

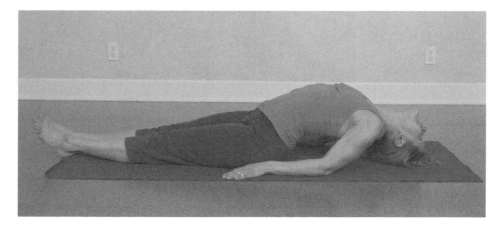

25. **Shoulder Stand

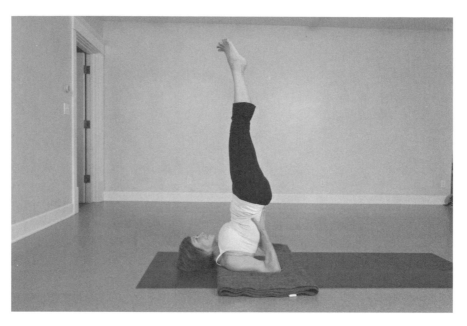

26. Bent Knee Twist (First Half Version)

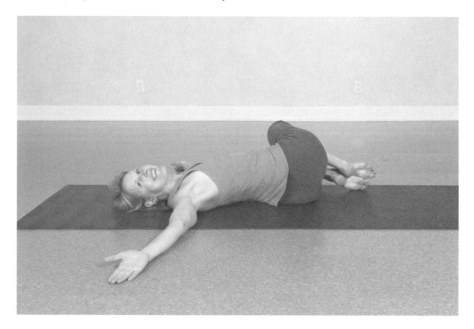

27. **Legs Up the Wall Pose

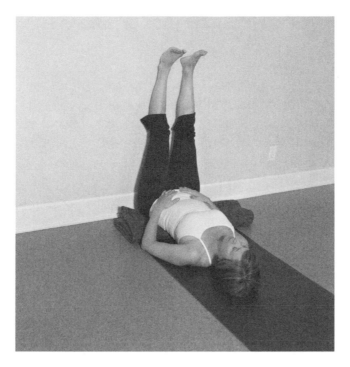

28. Supported Reclined Cobbler Pose

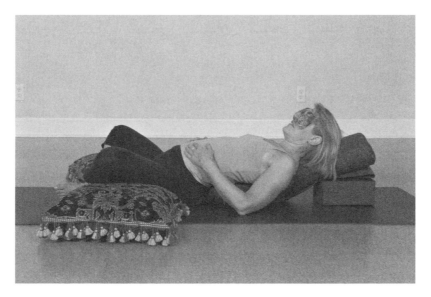

POSE DESCRIPTIONS FOR FIRST HALF INTERMEDIATE ROUTINE

I. CENTERING/CALMING BREATH (BELLY BREATH)

Setup

This breath can be performed either seated or lying down. Lie down on your back on your mat with your legs straight, or bend the knees if that is more comfortable for the low back. Another option is to sit in a chair with a solid seat that will allow you to sit with a long spine. Let your body relax and place your hands on your low belly.

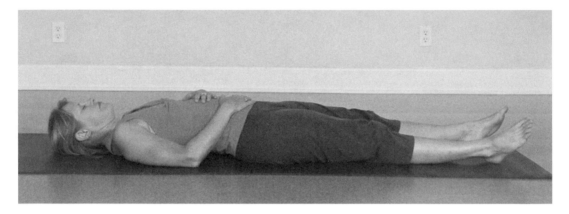

Movement

Breathe fully and deeply into your abdominal region, visualizing the prana (life force energy) filling your belly and creating the loving, open space for life. On the exhalations, visualize stress, defeating thoughts, frustration, etc. all leaving the body. Feel the muscles relax and get heavy with each exhalation. On the inhalations, invite the prana into every cell of your body and feel your hands rise with your breath. Let the gentle rhythm of your breath take you deeper and deeper into relaxation. Set an intention related to your fertility journey. This can be as simple as "I intend to get pregnant and have a beautiful, healthy baby." It can also be something like, "I intend to be kind to myself in this process of trying to conceive." Continue this breathing until you feel calm, and the breath is smooth and even. Ideally, the inhale and exhale should be either equal in length, or the exhale should be a little longer. Allow there to be a bit of a pause at the end of the exhale, and the end of the inhale, before you start the next breath. This "space" is perhaps the most important part of the breath. Try at least 12 full inhales and exhales, but feel free to do more if your mind hasn't calmed after 12 breaths.

Why Do This?

This centering/calming breathing technique helps the body and mind relax. The deep, conscious breaths activate the parasympathetic nervous system which promotes relaxation. This is a wonderful way to begin the practice or a technique that can be used any time you need to de-stress.

✿ POSES LYING ON YOUR BACK

2. KNEES TO CHEST

Setup

Now practice incorporating a simple movement with slow, conscious breathing. Bend your knees, and take your feet up off the floor. Place your hands on your knees.

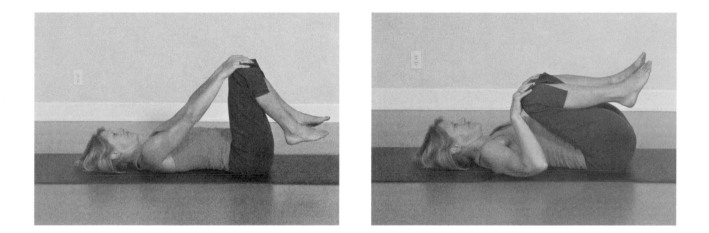

Movement

On an exhale, bring your knees gently toward your chest; don't hug them in, just gently draw them in. On an inhale, push the knees gently away as far as your arms can comfortably reach. The feet will remain off of the floor. Repeat the movement 5 to 8 more times. The focus should be mostly on the breath, rather than on the movement. Move slowly, using the whole exhale to bring the knees toward your chest, and the whole inhale to straighten your arms again.

Why Do This?

This simple movement allows you to get used to integrating the breath with movement. See if you can make your focus be on the breath, and just let the movement happen, with the breath leading the way. This is a very different approach than we use for most kinds of exercise—usually we are thinking about the activity or movement we need to do, and the breath just has to keep up. As a yoga practice, try to make it mostly about the breath, with the movement just following. This pose releases tension in the low back and sacrum, and helps clear bloating from the digestive tract.

3. COMING UP

Setup

To prepare for the next set of poses, bend your knees and roll onto your right side. Take a breath or two on your right side.

Movement

Use both hands to gently press yourself back up to a seated position.

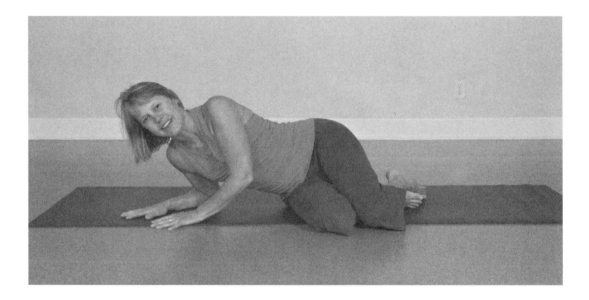

Why Do This?

Rolling to the side and pressing the floor inhibits tension in the neck and lower back. Rolling to the right side keeps the heart on top, so that you don't compress the heart (which is located on the left side). It also keeps the pulse regular, and frees up the breath through the left nostril, which promotes relaxation.

POSES ON HANDS AND KNEES

4. CAT-COW

Setup

Come onto your hands and knees with your wrists underneath your shoulders and your knees underneath your hips. Spread the fingers wide apart from each other. Your knees should be 4–6 inches apart. If this position bothers your knees, you can try folding a blanket and placing it underneath your knees for extra padding.

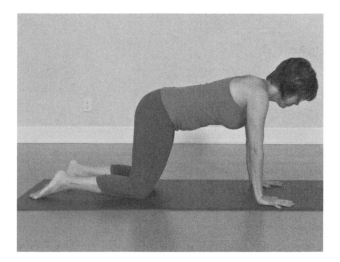

Movement

On an inhale, tilt your tailbone up and arch your back. Look forward and draw the shoulders back away from the ears. Keep your core engaged as you arch the back. On an exhale, tilt your tailbone down toward the floor and round your spine. Press the shoulder blades up toward the ceiling. Let your head and neck feel heavy. Repeat at least 5 times, initiating each movement at the tailbone. Allow the movement to follow the breath.

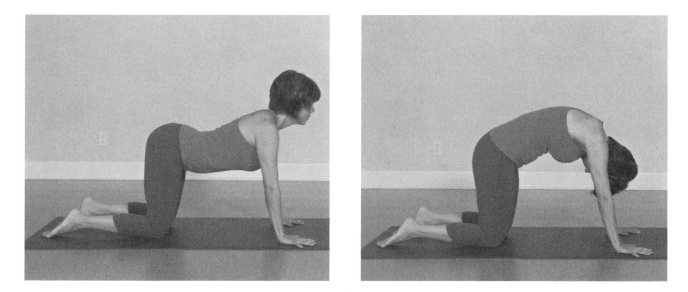

Why Do This?

Cat-cow warms up all of the muscles in the back and allows tension in the neck and shoulders to release. It also opens the major energy channels in the front and back of the body. The pelvic movements bring blood flow and energy through the pelvis.

5. CAT-COW CIRCLES

Setup

Setup is the same as for Cat-Cow.

Movement

Circle the hips and ribcage around to the right, bending the elbows as much as you need to. This is a very free-form movement, so just do what feels good to your body. You may get some forward-and-back movement as well as the circling. Don't forget to use deep, full breaths while performing these circles. After a few breaths, switch directions.

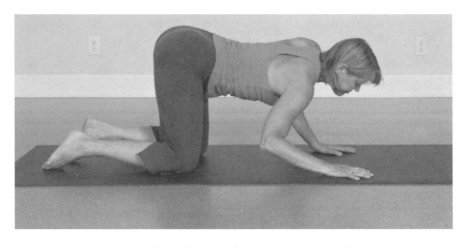

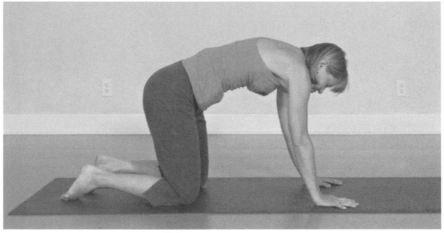

Why Do This?

The circling motion releases tension in the pelvis, ribcage and shoulders. We are taking the torso through a range of motion that most of us don't experience in our regular daily lives, so it encourages us to release physical and emotional patterns where we may be "stuck."

6. DOWNWARD FACING DOG

Setup

From the hands and knees position, take an inhale and engage the muscles of the arms. Relax the space between your shoulder blades.

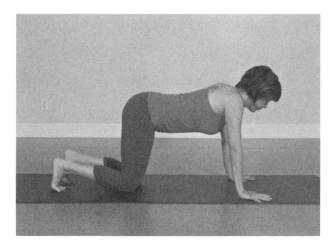
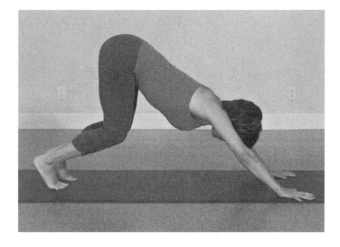

Movement

Exhale, curl your toes under and lift your knees off of the floor. Lift the hips, and draw the low belly up and back. Press strongly through the hands, and draw energy from the hands up the arms. Take a peek back at your feet and be sure they are "sitting-bones-width" distance apart (about 4–6 inches apart) and parallel. Keep the under-sides of the arms lifting away from the floor. Your heels may or may not touch the floor. If you feel a lot of stretch in your hamstrings, bend the knees slightly, allowing the back to lengthen. Stay here for 5 to 8 breaths feeling

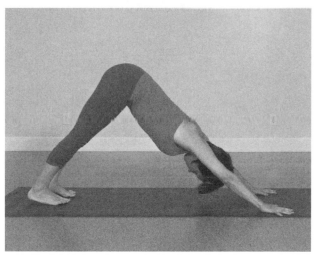

the whole body stretch and lengthen. Then inhale, bend the knees, and return to the hands and knees position. **Don't do this pose for an extended length of time if you are on your period.**

Why Do This?

Downward dog is a full body stretch that is good for the whole body. It is also a partial inversion which is beneficial for the circulatory system as well as for the endocrine system. It tones the abdominal muscles and can help regulate the menstrual cycle. However, you should not do this pose for an extended period of time during the main flow days of your period.

7. PRAYER POSE (CHILD'S POSE)

Setup

From the hands and knees position, take the knees wide apart and sit the hips back onto the heels. Keep the toes together. Bring the forehead to the floor, and reach the arms forward with the palms facing down. If it isn't comfortable to bring the forehead all the way to the floor, you can stack the hands one on top of the other, and rest the forehead on the hands, or rest the forehead on a block or a folded blanket. Let the toes release.

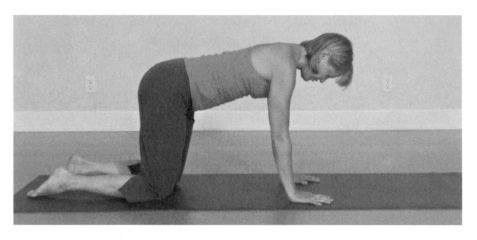

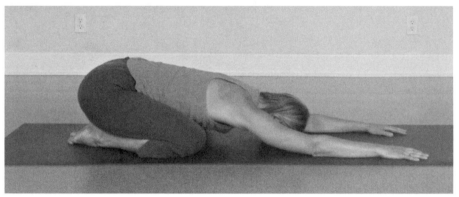

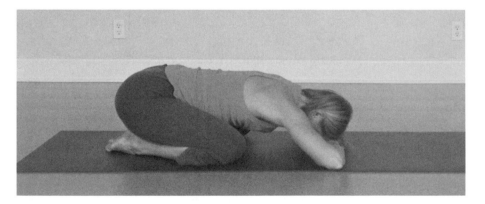

Movement

Prayer pose is a resting pose, so in the standard version of prayer pose, you are resting here, rather than moving. To come up from prayer pose, just walk the hands back in toward the body, and come up slowly.

8. VARIATION (CHILD'S POSE)

In prayer pose, reach the arms back along the outside of the calves, rather than reaching forward.

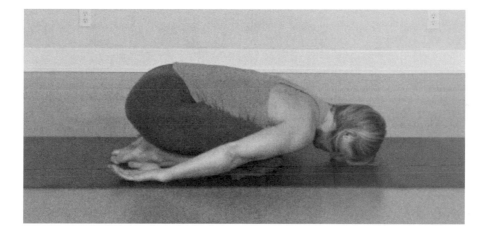

Why Do This?

Prayer pose is a resting pose that is known for its calming effect, which is partly due to resting the forehead down. It also stretches and relaxes the hips and low back.

9. KNEE-DOWN LUNGE

Setup

From prayer pose, walk your hands back in toward your body, raising your torso.

Movement

Step your right foot forward between your hands and curl your back toes under so you are pressing the ball of the left foot into the floor. Squeeze the legs in towards an imaginary midline down the center of your body and place both hands on your right thigh. Stay here or reach your arms over your head while relaxing your shoulders. Take 5 full breaths here. Retrace your steps carefully until you are back to a tabletop position on your hands and knees. Repeat steps on the left side.

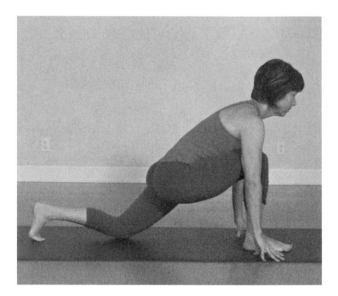

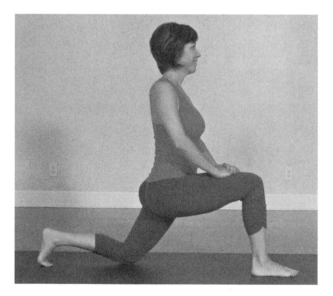

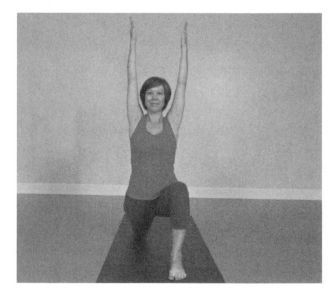

Why Do This?

This pose tones the abdominal organs including the reproductive organs. It opens the quadriceps, which allows more circulation and energy to flow into the pelvic area.

10. GROIN STRETCH (LIZARD LUNGE)

Setup

Begin on your hands and knees in a tabletop position.

Movement

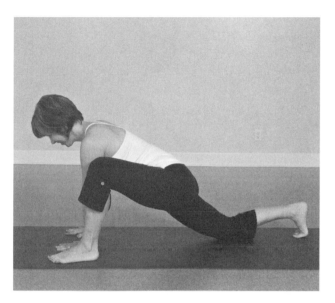

Bring your left foot forward, keeping your right knee down on the floor. Walk your front foot out slightly to the left, making sure your knee stays over your ankle. Place both hands to the inside of the front foot. Walk the hands forward and place your forearms on the floor or on blocks if the floor is too challenging. Try to keep your spine elongated; the tendency will be for the back to round. Breathe into your hips and groins. You may want to lift the back knee if that feels appropriate. This will deepen the stretch. Stay in this pose for 5 to 8 breaths. Repeat on the second side.

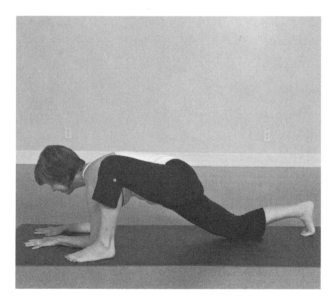

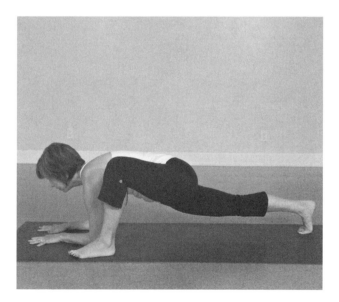

Why Do This?

This pose opens the hips and inner thighs and tones the abdominal organs.

11. PIGEON POSE

Setup

Begin on your hands and knees in a tabletop position.

Movement

Slide your left knee toward your left hand, bringing the left foot in front of the right hip. Your left knee should be on the floor about 2 inches to the left of the hip bone. Walk your right leg straight back behind you allowing the top of the foot to rest on the floor. Square your hips forward and come down onto your forearms. If you find that you are collapsing onto the hip on the bent-knee side, place a blanket underneath the buttock (see photo).

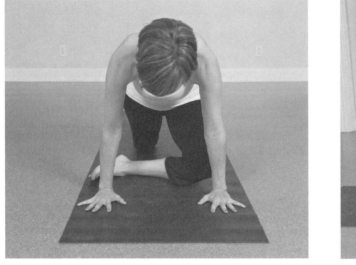
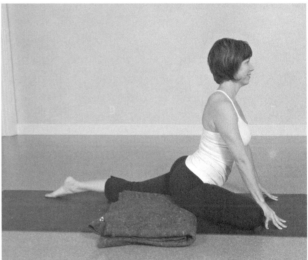

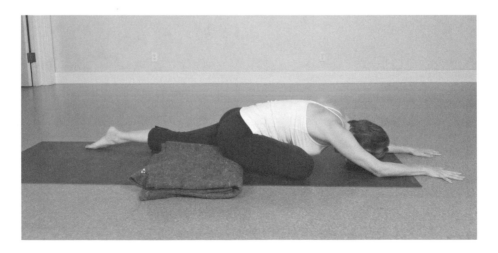

12. VARIATION: TWIST IN PIGEON POSE

After 5 breaths, add a twist to your Pigeon Pose by taking your right hand across onto your left knee. Allow your right forearm to rest down on the mat. Bring your left hand around behind you, resting the palm on your sacrum. Twist toward the left, taking care not to collapse into the front shoulder. Move the neck around gently until you find a place where it feels comfortable. The neck should feel like an extension of the rest of the spine. Take 5 breaths in the twist.

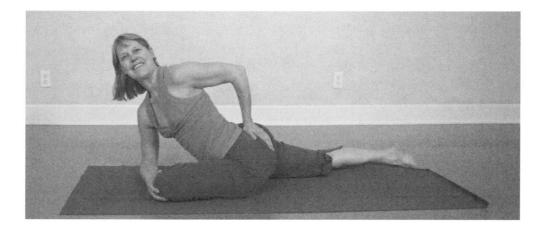

After completing the pose on the left side, curl your back toes under and press into your hands. Lift your hips up and come into downward facing dog. Bring the right knee forward and do the second side of the pose. After completing the second side of the pose, curl your back toes under and press into your hands. Lift your hips up and come into downward facing dog. Walk your feet up to meet your hands and come up to a standing position at the front of your mat.

Why Do This?

Pigeon pose is a great hip opener that stretches the outer hip rotators, groins, psoas and thighs as well as the abdomen. Adding the twist stimulates the abdominal organs and stretches the shoulders, neck and back.

❀ STANDING POSES

13. WARRIOR 2 POSE WITH EAGLE ARMS

Setup

Turn to face the long side of your mat. Step your feet about 3 ½ to 4 feet apart. Turn your right foot out 90 degrees so that the outer edge of your foot aligns with the right side of your mat. Keep your left foot pointing straight ahead or turn it in slightly, and align the arch of the back foot with the heel of the front foot.

Movement

Bend your right knee toward 90 degrees, keeping your knee over your ankle. Bring your arms in front of you with the elbows bent to a 90 degree angle. Bring your right arm underneath your left arm allowing the backs of the hands to touch or bringing the palms together. Try to keep your elbows at shoulder height. Breathe into tension or tightness in the mid to upper back. Take 5 to 8 breaths in the pose. Come out of the pose slowly by first unwinding the arms. Pivot the feet so the left foot turns out 90 degrees and the right foot points straight ahead or turns in slightly. Repeat steps above on the left side.

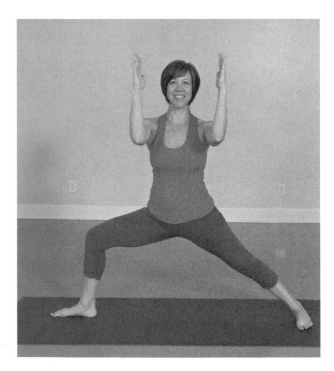 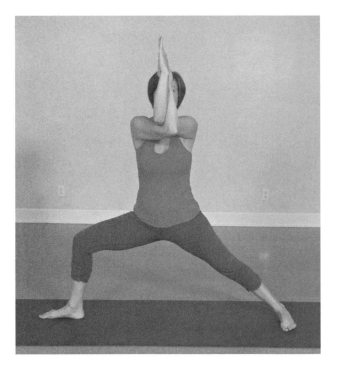

Why Do This?

This pose releases tension in the shoulders and tones the abdominal organs.

14.   SIDE ANGLE POSE

Setup

Facing the long side of your mat, step your feet about 3 ½ to 4 feet apart. Turn your right foot out 90 degrees so that the outer edge of your foot aligns with the side of your mat. Keep your left foot pointing straight ahead or turn it in slightly.

Movement

Bend your right knee toward 90 degrees keeping your knee over your ankle. Lean to the right and place your right forearm just above your knee. Place your left hand on your waist and turn your torso toward the sky. Stay here or extend your left arm over your head, keeping the bicep over the ear with the palm facing down. Anchor this forward movement by firmly pressing the outer edge of the back foot into the floor. Take 5–8 breaths. To come up, press down through the feet and legs and bring your torso back up to vertical on an inhale. Pivot the feet so the left foot turns out to 90 degrees and the right foot points straight ahead or turns in slightly. Repeat steps above on the left side.

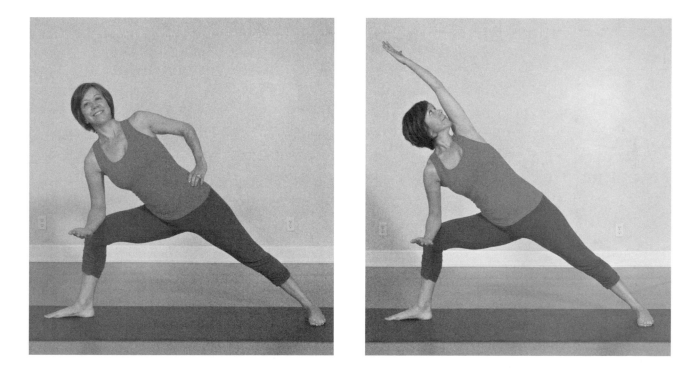

Why Do This?

Side Angle pose tones the pelvic organs and increases circulation and energy flow through the entire torso region. It can also help with menstrual problems.

15. TRIANGLE POSE

Setup

Facing the long side of your mat, step your feet about 3 ½ to 4 feet apart. Turn your right foot out to the right about 90 degrees, and align the arch of the back foot with the heel of the front foot. Raise your arms parallel to the floor with the palms facing down.

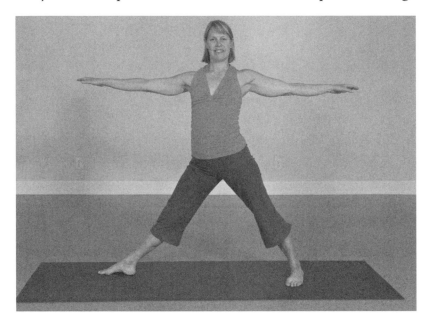

Movement

Exhale and reach out through the right arm, extending your torso forward over the right leg. Bend from the hip joint, not the waist; try to keep the underneath side of the waist long.

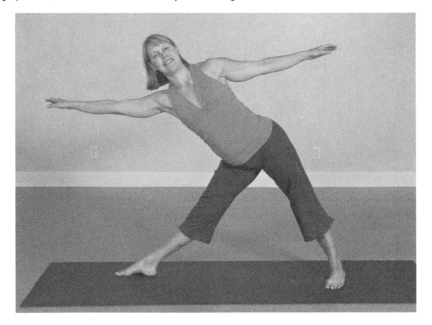

Let your right hand come onto your leg, just letting it rest wherever it comes naturally after reaching out through the right arm. It will likely come to the shin, but possibly to the ankle, or even above the knee joint (don't rest it on the knee joint, though). (Option: use a block underneath the hand, rather than resting the hand on the leg. This adds stability).

Anchor this forward movement by firmly pressing the outer edge of the back foot into the floor. Rotate the ribs toward the ceiling, keeping both the upper and lower sides of the torso equally long. Reach your left arm toward the ceiling, in line with the tops of your shoulders. You can look down at the left hand, or up at the ceiling, or look to the side. If the neck feels uncomfortable, move it around gently and see if you can find a place where it feels in better alignment. Take 5 to 8 deep breaths. To come up, inhale and press through the front foot. You could imagine that someone is pulling on your top arm to bring you back up to standing. Reverse the feet and repeat for the same length of time on the second side.

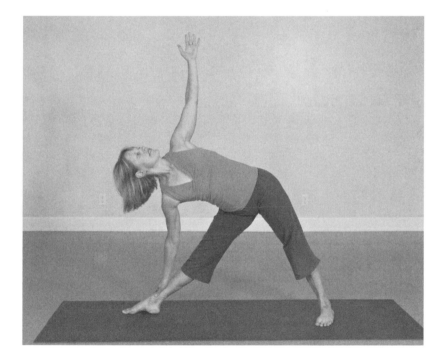

Why Do This?

Triangle pose creates a lot of space in the torso, improving circulation and energy flow through the internal organs and glands.

16. HALF-MOON BALANCE POSE

Setup

Stand in the center of your mat facing the short edge of the mat. Place your feet hip-width (4–6 inches) apart. Step forward with your right foot and take your weight onto your right foot as you allow the right knee to bend a little. Reach your right hand forward, and bring it down to the floor. It should be at least 12 inches in front of the foot, about in line with the little-toe side of the right foot. (Option: use a block underneath the hand; this is easier to reach than the floor).

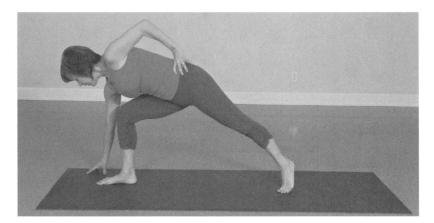

Movement

Begin to straighten your right leg, while lifting the left leg parallel (or a little above parallel) to the floor. Reach back through the left heel to keep the raised leg reaching back strongly. Be careful not to lock or hyperextend the standing knee. Check that the kneecap is aligned over the big toe, or even the 2nd toe (not to the inside of the big toe). Most of the weight should be on the foot, not the hand. Rotate your upper torso to the left. *Easiest:* Keep the left hand on the left hip and the eyes gazing down toward the floor near your right hand. *More advanced*: Open the left arm up toward the ceiling, and turn the head to look toward the left. Stay in this position for 3 or more breaths. Then perform the pose standing on the left foot for the same length of time.

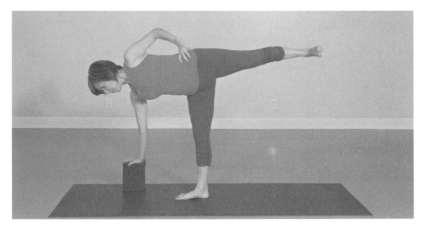

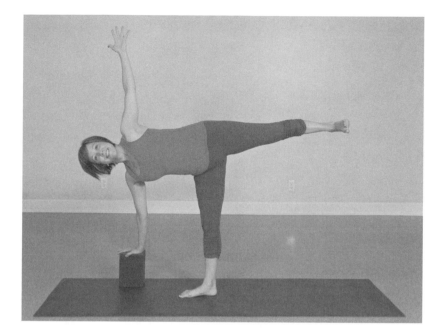

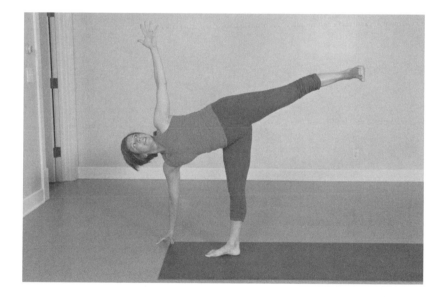

Why Do This?

Half-moon balance pose creates a lot of space in the torso, improving circulation and energy flow through the internal organs and glands. It also requires us to keep our focus in the present moment.

17. WIDE STANDING FORWARD BEND WITH IMMUNE BOOSTER

Setup

Stand with your feet about 3 feet apart, facing one of the long edges of your mat. Take your hands on your hips. Make sure your feet are parallel to each other.

Movement

On an exhale, lean the torso forward from the hip joints. You can bend the knees slightly if your low back feels any strain as you come forward. Release your hands onto the floor directly below your shoulders (or place a block here). Allow the head to release down toward the floor, and take a few breaths here. Then reach the hands behind the back and interweave the fingers together. The backs of the hands should be facing the ceiling, palms toward the back. Keep a slight bend in the elbows, rather than allowing them to hyper-extend. On an inhale, bring the arms up away from the back, and lower again on the exhale. Repeat several times. Then release the hands back down to the floor.

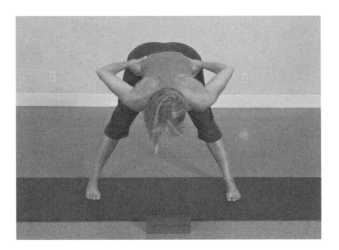

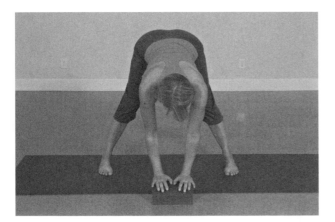

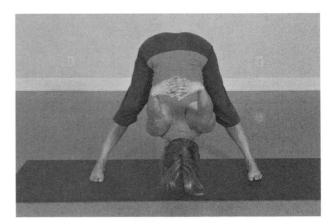

Coming up to Standing

Walk the feet towards each other until they are 6 inches or so apart. Bend the knees slightly, let the head and arms hang, and slowly roll up to standing one vertebra at a time. The chin should stay tucked to the chest until you are all the way back to vertical; bring the head up last.

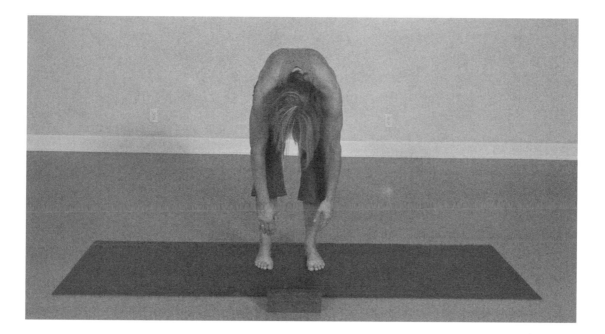

Why Do This?

In addition to the obvious stretch of the hamstrings, forward bends support the endocrine system and help bring hormonal balance to the body. They also tone the organs in the abdominal area, and are calming to the central nervous system. Forward bends raise the yin energy in the body. Taking the arms up and away from the back, with the hands clasped, is an immune system booster, in addition to opening the shoulders.

✦ SUPINE POSES

18. **MOVING COBRA

Setup

Lie on your belly with the forehead resting on the mat. Clasp your hands behind your back.

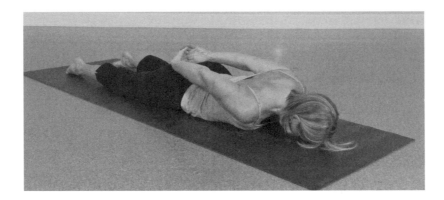

Movement

On an inhale, raise the head and shoulders up away from the floor. Keep the eyes looking down at the floor, to keep the back of the neck long. Exhale, and lower your head and shoulders back down on the floor. Repeat 4–6 times. **Don't do this pose if you are on your period.**

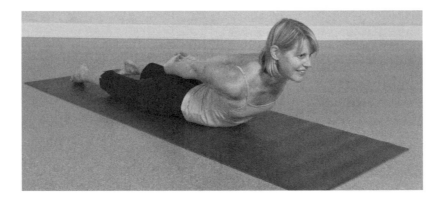

Why Do This?

This pose is very stimulating, cleansing and nourishing for the ovaries and abdominal organs. When you rise up, you compress the belly and squeeze the blood out of the organs. As you lower the body back down, the organs receive a fresh blood supply.

19.   **BOW POSE

Setup

Lie on your belly with the forehead resting on the mat. Bend your knees, bringing your heels as close as you can to your buttocks. Reach back with your hands and take hold of your ankles. Place a folded blanket under the pubic bone if it is uncomfortable.

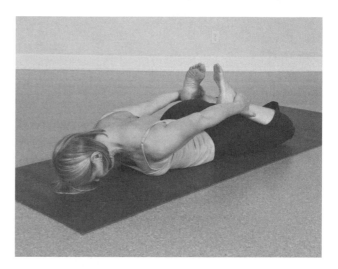

Movement

Inhale and strongly lift your heels away from your buttocks and, at the same time, lift your thighs away from the floor. The head and upper torso will also rise up as you pull back and up with your heels. Draw the tops of the shoulders away from your ears and lengthen the back of the neck. Look straight ahead (not up) to keep the neck lengthening. Make sure your knees are no wider than hip width, i.e., you are pulling straight back, not out to the sides. If you find breathing difficult in this position, try to breathe more into the back of your torso, rather than into the belly. If you have any low back discomfort, try a lower position, or come out of the pose and rest. After a few breaths in bow pose, release on an exhale, and lie quietly for a few breaths. You can repeat the pose once or twice more. *Tips:* If you have trouble lifting your thighs away from the floor, you can give your legs a little upward boost by lying with your thighs supported on a rolled-up blanket. If it isn't possible for you to hold your ankles directly, just practice Cobra pose until you can easily reach the ankles with your hands. **Don't do this pose if you are on your period.

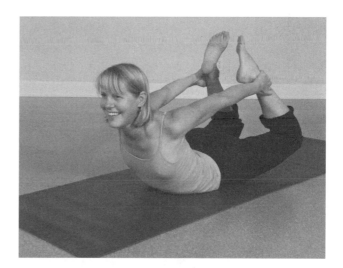

Why Do This?

This pose is very stimulating for the ovaries and abdominal organs. When you raise the torso while resting on the belly, you compress the low belly which contains the reproductive organs. This stimulates circulation and energy flow, and the organs receive a fresh, nourishing blood supply.

20. **LOCUST

Setup

Lie on your belly with the forehead resting on the floor. Make your hands into
fists and take them underneath your body,
palms facing up. Place them so that the
middle joints of the fingers touch the pubic
bone, and the thumbs touch each other.
Make sure the forearms are to the inside of
the front hip bones (ASIS bones), and not
underneath the bones, or this will be very
uncomfortable.

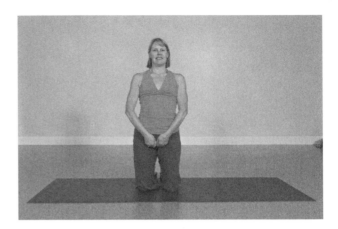

Movement

On the inhale, raise the right leg up away from the floor. Be careful not to raise the hip or
tilt the pelvis—just raise the leg, without bending the knee. Keep the eyes looking down at
the floor, to keep the back of the neck long. Exhale, and lower the leg. Continue, alternating between the right and left leg. Do a total of 4 lifts for each leg. **Don't do this pose if
you are on your period**. *More advanced:* Try raising both legs together and holding them
up for 3 breaths. Then lower the legs and rest.

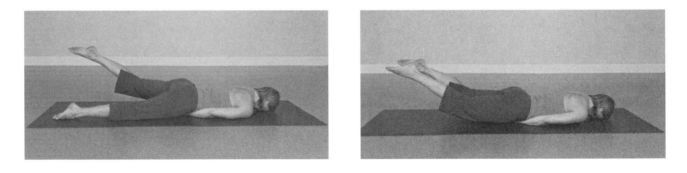

Why Do This?

This pose is very stimulating for the ovaries and abdominal organs. When you raise the leg,
the fists compress the area of the low belly containing the ovaries and uterus. This stimulates circulation and energy flow, and as you lower the leg, the glands and organs receive
a fresh blood supply.

21. PRAYER POSE VARIATION

Setup

Draw the hips back toward the heels. Move hips gently side-to-side in prayer pose to release the low back. Take a few resting breaths here.

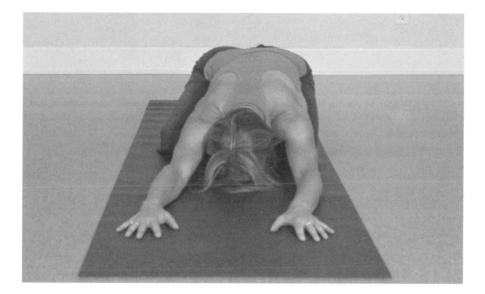

✤ MORE POSES LYING ON YOUR BACK

22. **PELVIC TILTS WITH PELVIC FLOOR CONTRACTIONS

Setup

Lie down on your back with your knees bent and your feet on the floor, hip-width (4–6 inches) apart. Let your palms rest on the floor on either side of your hips.

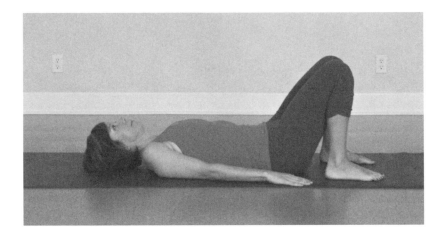

Movement

On an exhale, *gently* tilt the pelvis to press the low back down into the floor. At the same time, contract and lift the pelvic floor muscles. (See Pose #26 in the First Half Basic Routine for more description on how to do this). On an inhale, release the pelvic floor and let the low back come up again. Repeat 4–6 times. **Don't do this pose if you are on your period.**

Why Do This?

While there are versions of this which are used for core strengthening, that is not our purpose here. We are using this pose to create a gentle rocking of the pelvis. This encourages blood and energy flow, and releases tension and stagnation in the pelvis. For this purpose, press the low back down *gently*, trying not to engage the abdominal muscles any more than necessary to get the action to happen. Pelvic floor lifts help tone the PC muscle, and increase blood flow to the pelvic organs.

23. **BRIDGE POSE

Setup

Setup is the same as for Pelvic Tilts.

Movement

On an inhale, press both feet and hands into the floor and lift the hips straight up toward the sky. Try to bring your shoulder blades toward each other while gently pressing the back of the head into the floor. You can stay here pressing your hands into the floor or clasp your hands underneath your back. With your hands clasped, draw the wrists towards the floor. Take 5 to 8 breaths. To come out of the pose, on an inhale, take your arms up past your head on the floor. Exhale and lower your body down slowly, from the upper back to the low back and hips. Try to roll down one vertebra at a time. **Don't do this pose if you are on your period.**

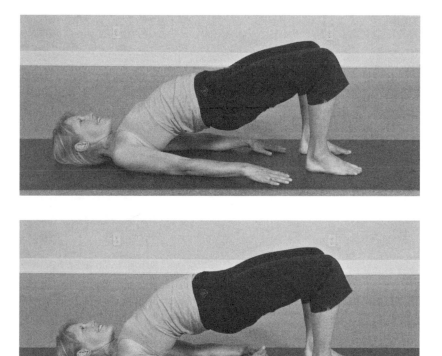

Why Do This?

Bridge pose releases tension in the upper back and brings energy and vitality to the reproductive organs. It is also releases tension in the neck and shoulders, and helps to regulate the thyroid gland.

24. FISH POSE

Setup

With your hands palms down on either side of you, tuck your forearms and elbows up close to the sides of your torso.

Movement

Press your forearms and elbows firmly against the floor. With an inhale, lift your upper torso and head up and well away from the floor. Then gently release your head back onto the floor, arching the neck so that the crown of the head rests on the floor. Use your hands and forearms to help reduce the amount of weight on your head. Stay for a few breaths, breathing smoothly. With an exhalation lower your torso and head to the floor. Draw your thighs up toward your belly and squeeze gently. **Don't do this pose if you have had a neck injury or if you experience neck pain as you come into the pose.**

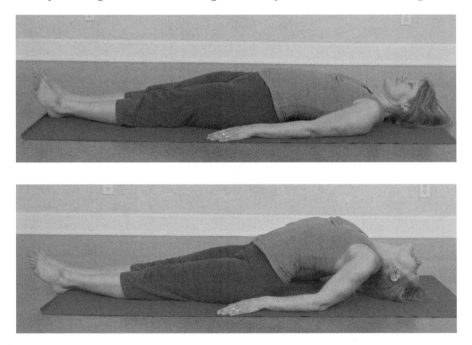

Why Do This?

A traditional yoga text calls Fish Pose the "destroyer of all diseases." Some of the key benefits for fertility include:

- Stretches the deep hip flexors (psoas), releasing tension in the pelvic area.
- Stretches the muscles (intercostals) between the ribs, which improves your ability to breathe deeply.
- Stretches and stimulates the organs of the belly and throat, and boosts the immune system.
- Helps to regulate the thyroid and parathyroid glands, which control metabolism.

25. **SHOULDER STAND

Setup

Place a folded blanket on one end of your mat. Lie down on your back with your knees bent and your feet on the floor, with the blanket underneath your upper back and shoulders, as shown in the photo. The shoulders will be about and an inch and a half below the clean fold of the blanket.

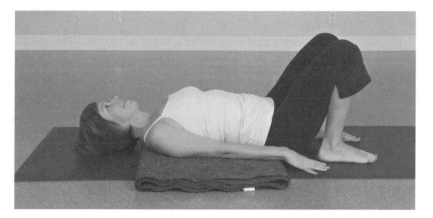

Movement

Draw your knees toward your chest and bring your hands underneath your hips as you lift your hips and legs off the floor. Support the weight of the hips with your hands and extend your legs straight up toward the ceiling. Keep your core engaged and the muscles in the legs activated. The weight should rest on the shoulders, NOT on the neck. If the weight is resting on the neck, add more folded blankets to your stack. Press up through the balls of the feet. Stay in the pose for up to 1 or 2 minutes. If you feel any discomfort in your neck or back, come out of the pose and rest on your back. Release the pose by slowly lowering the hips into the hands and bringing the feet back down on the floor. **Don't do this pose if you are on your period.**

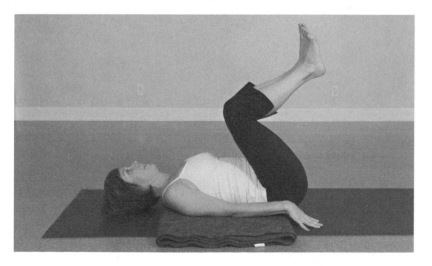

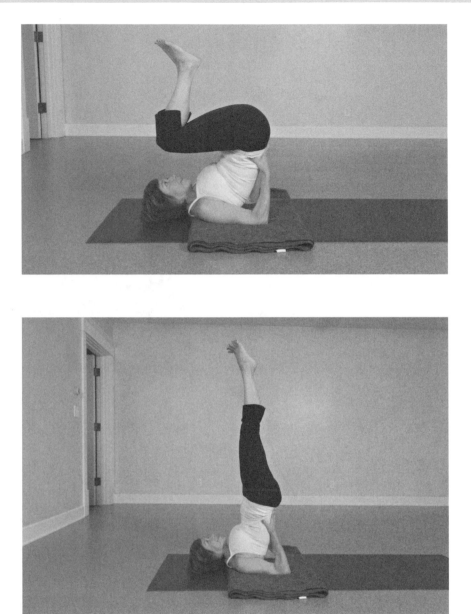

Why Do This?

This pose helps stimulate the thyroid gland and abdominal organs. It has a calming effect on the brain and can help reduce stress and fatigue as well as alleviate insomnia. Shoulder stand stretches the neck and shoulders and tones the buttocks and legs.

26. BENT KNEE TWIST (FIRST HALF VERSION)

Setup

Lie on your back on your mat with your knees bent and feet on the floor. Take the feet to the outer edges of your yoga mat. The feet will be about two feet apart. Now, take the arms out to the sides like a "T," with your palms facing up.

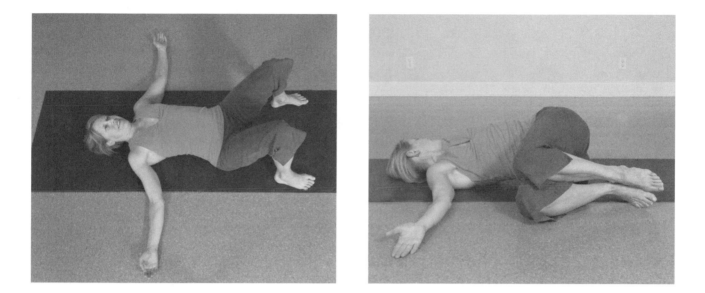

Movement

Lift the hips and shift them slightly toward the left. Then allow the knees to drop slowly over toward the right. Pick up the left knee and place it on top of the right knee. The knees can come all the way to the floor, if your ribcage and back allow. You may find a trade-off between the knees coming to the floor, and the opposite shoulder coming off the ground. In this case, allow the knees to come down, and then try to release the shoulder toward the floor, as you can. Turn the head to look back toward the left palm. Take 5 to 8 slow, even breaths. On an inhale, bring the knees back to center, and do the twist to the second side.

Why Do This?

Twists like this are cleansing and rejuvenating for the organs (such as the uterus and intestines) and glands (such as the ovaries) in the abdominal area. As you twist, the blood is squeezed out of those organs and glands like wringing out a sponge. As you come out of the twist, a fresh nourishing blood supply is delivered to them.

COMING UP

Setup

To prepare for the next set of poses, bend your knees and roll onto your right side. Take a breath or two on your right side.

Movement

Use both hands to gently press yourself back up to a seated position.

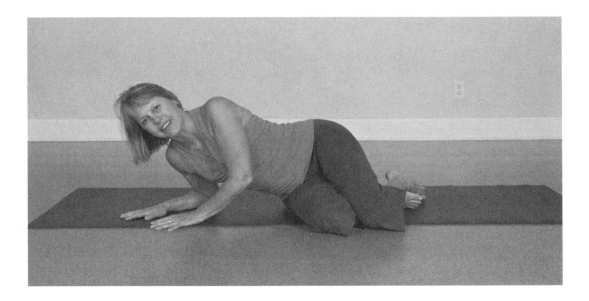

Why Do This?

Rolling to the side and pressing the floor inhibits tension in the neck and lower back. Rolling to the right side keeps the heart on top, so that you don't compress the heart (which is located on the left side). It also keeps the pulse regular, and frees up the breath through the left nostril, which promotes relaxation.

🪷 RELAXATION POSES

27.   **LEGS UP THE WALL POSE (WITH VARIATIONS)

Setup

Do this pose at a clear space of wall, where you have room to take your legs straight up the wall without bumping into anything. Before you start, put on warm clothes and socks, and have a blanket handy which you can pull over yourself once you get into the pose. Place your yoga mat lengthwise to the wall. Option: place a folded blanket on your mat next to the wall. This can be helpful if your hamstrings are tight or if your low back is uncomfortable in the pose.

Movement

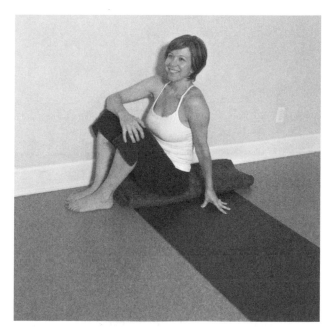

Start by sitting sideways at the wall, with your right hip just next to the wall and your knees bent. Place your left hand on the floor next to your left hip, and your right hand on the floor behind you. Lean back, taking some weight onto your hands. You might even come down onto your elbows. Next, swing your legs up the wall, so that your sitting bones end up fairly close to the wall. Once up, the hands can rest on the low belly, or on either side of you, about 12 inches away from the body, with the palms facing up toward the ceiling. **Don't do this pose if you are on your period.**

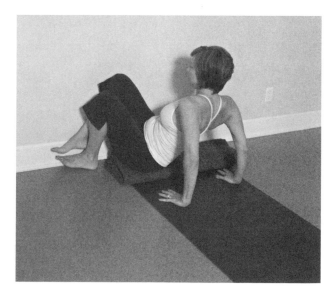

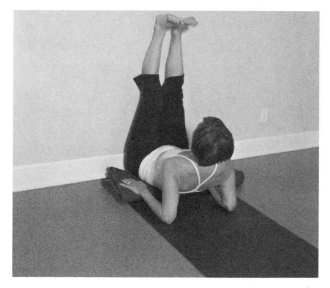

Variations

You can keep the legs a few inches apart on the wall, or try varying the leg position by taking them wider apart, or taking the soles of the feet together like cobbler pose at the wall. When you get ready to come out of the pose, draw the knees into the chest and roll onto your right side with your knees bent. Rest for a few breaths before using both hands to press up to a seated position.

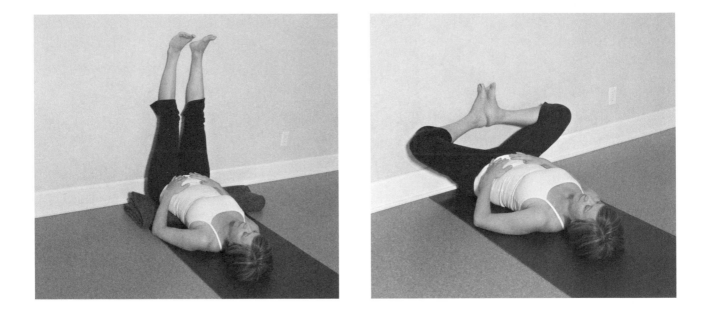

Why Do This?

This pose is one of the most powerful fertility-supporting yoga poses. The abdominal organs are nourished and revitalized when the blood from the feet and legs pools in the low belly. Toxins are removed from the bloodstream, as the blood flows into the lymph glands in the groin. The central nervous system is calmed and the endocrine system is regulated. It is a great pose to do just before bedtime, as it promotes restful sleep. This pose should be done daily for at least 5 minutes, during every part of the cycle except during menstruation.

28. RECLINED COBBLER POSE

Setup

Sit on the mat with your legs comfortably crossed and a bolster right behind you. Have the bolster close enough so that your sacrum is touching it. If you don't have a bolster, you can make one by rolling your yoga mat up in a folded blanket, and propping one end of this roll up on your block (see photo).

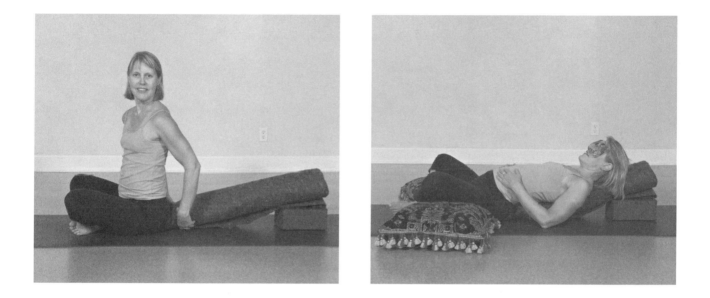

Movement

Bend your knees and bring the soles of the feet onto the mat and your hands on the mat next to your hips. Begin to slowly lower yourself back onto the bolster or blanket roll until your entire back and head are supported. Bring the soles of the feet together to touch, and slowly allow your knees to release toward the floor. You can place cushions or folded blankets under your thighs for additional support. Rest your hands on your belly, or allow them to gently rest by your sides, palms facing up. Stay in this pose for up to 10 minutes if time allows. Come out if the hips or knees feel any discomfort.

Why Do This?

This pose helps the abdomen, pelvis and lower back to relax. It allows for a gentle opening of the hips and can help alleviate menstrual pain. This pose is wonderful for helping the apana energy flow downwards, especially during menstruation.

Yoga for Fertility: Routines for the Second Half of Your Cycle

YOGA FOR FERTILITY: SECOND HALF BASIC ROUTINE

The following sequence of basic fertility yoga poses are ideally performed after ovulation up until the onset of your period. *(Once you have your period, you can do the Routine for Your Period in Chapter 6.)* The poses in this routine can also be performed safely if conception has occurred. After month 3 of your pregnancy, you may wish to perform a prenatal sequence, which will modify poses for optimal comfort and safety as you progress in your pregnancy. See Chapter 6 for a Prenatal Yoga Sequence that can be used during your first trimester.

SUMMARY FLOW OF SECOND HALF BASIC ROUTINE

Note: A double asterisk ** means you should not practice this pose during the main flow days of your period.

1. **Centering/Calming Breath (Belly Breath)**

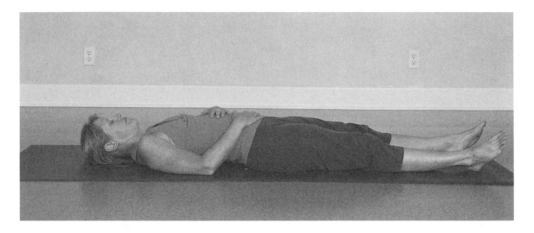

2. **Knees to Chest**

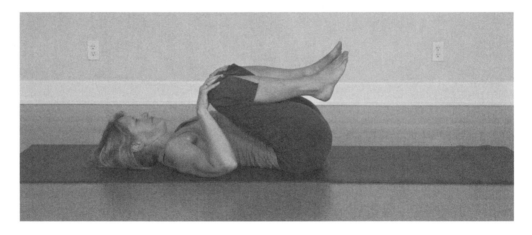

3. **Moving Bridge**

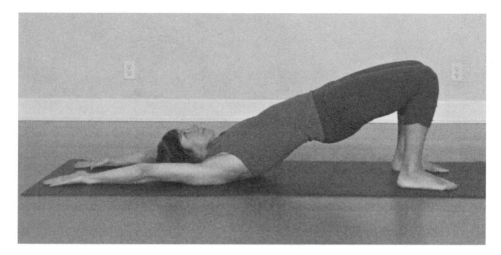

4. ****Supported Bridge**

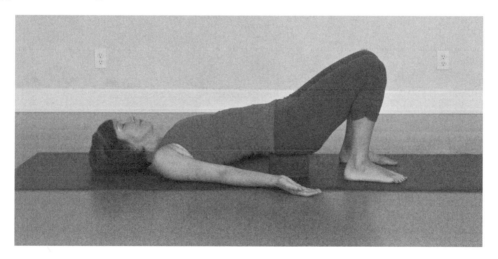

5. **Sacrum Circles**

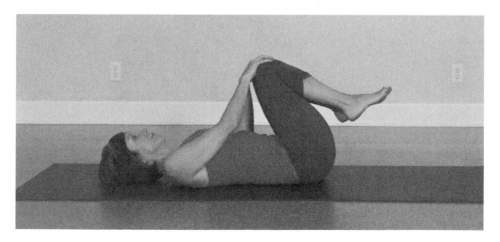

6. **Outer Hip Stretch (#4 Pose)**

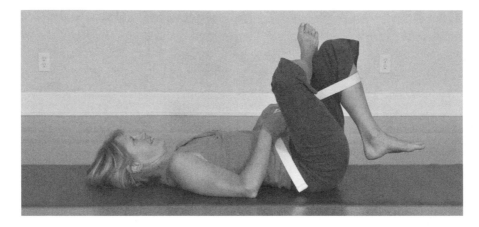

7. **Happy Baby Pose**

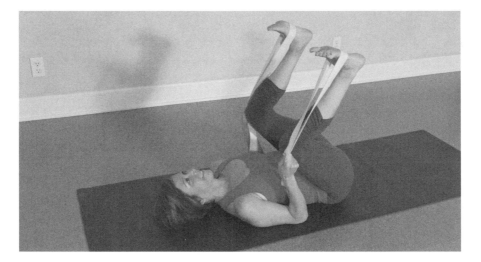

8. **Pelvic Tilts**

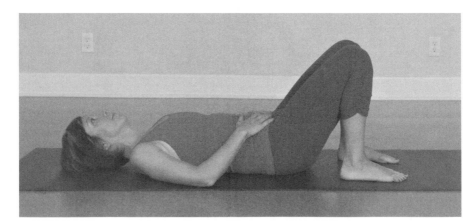

9. **Bent Knee Twist (2nd Half Version)**

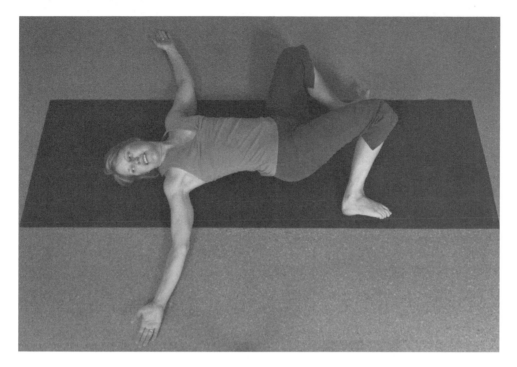

10. **Coming Up**

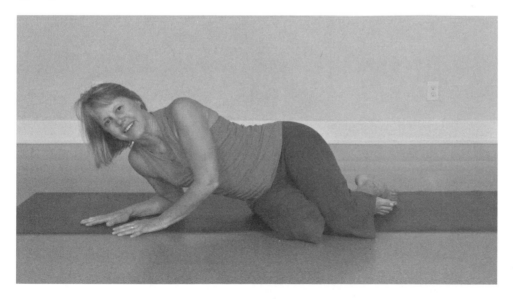

11. Cat-Cow

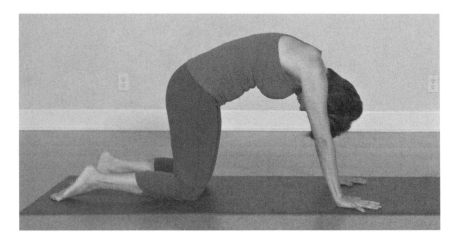

12. Cat-Cow Circles

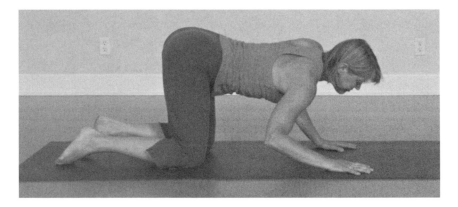

13. Prayer Pose (Child's Pose)

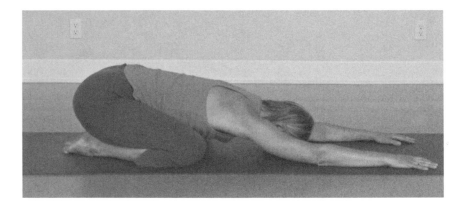

14. ****Downward Facing Dog**

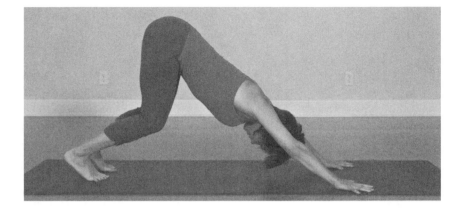

15. **Prayer Pose (Child's Pose)**

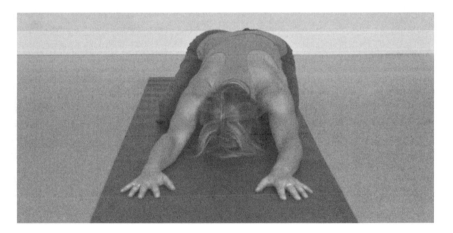

16. **Knee-Down Lunge**

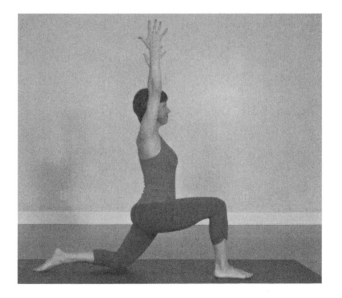

17. Mountain Pose

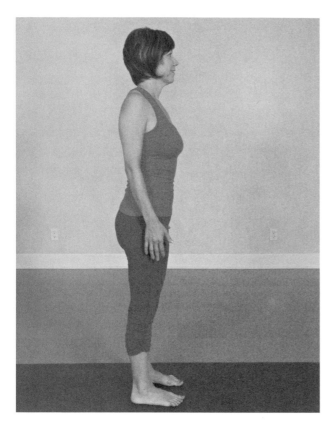

18. Tree Pose

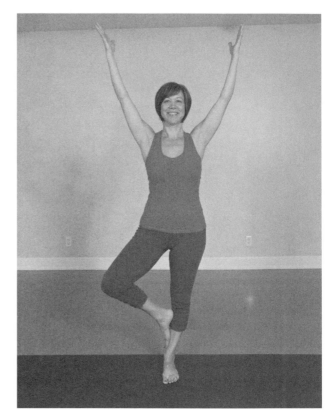

19. Side Angle Pose

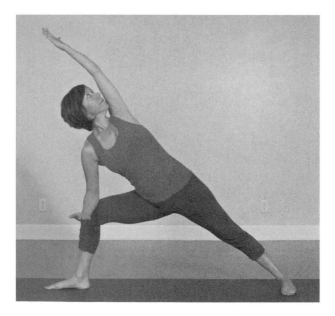

20. Squat Pose and Variations

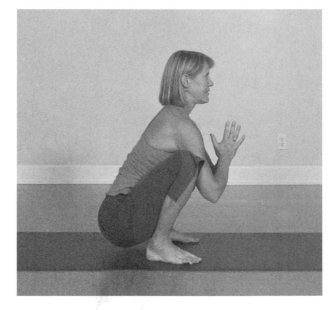

21. "Chicken Wing" Shoulder Stretch

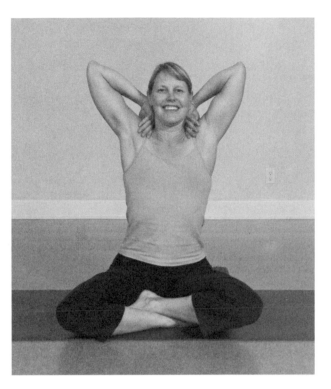

22. Seated Wide-Leg Straddle and Variation

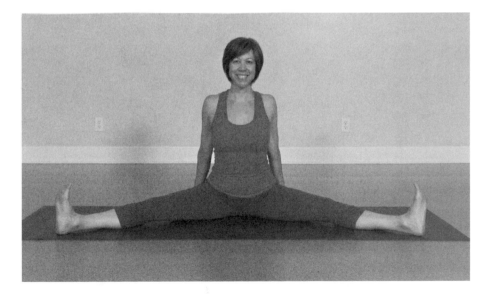

23. **Cobbler Pose**

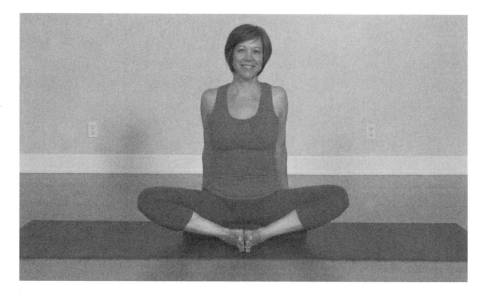

24. ****Legs Up the Wall Pose**

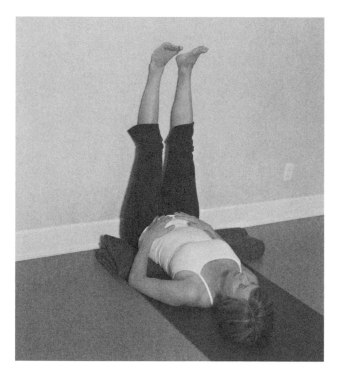

25. Corpse Pose

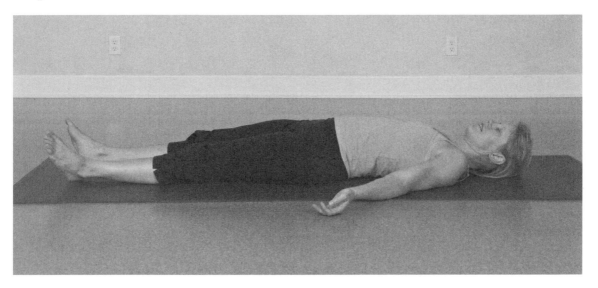

POSE DESCRIPTIONS FOR SECOND HALF BASIC ROUTINE

1. CENTERING/CALMING BREATH (BELLY BREATH)

Setup

This breath can be performed either seated or lying down. Lie on your back on your mat with your legs straight, or bend the knees if that is more comfortable for the low back. Another option is to sit in a chair with a solid seat that will allow you to sit with a long spine. Let your body relax and place your hands on your low belly.

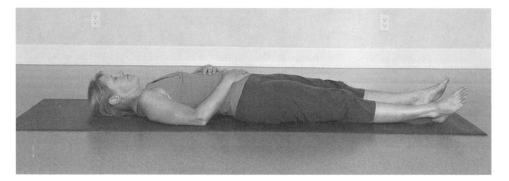

Movement

Breathe fully and deeply into your abdominal region, visualizing the prana (life force energy) filling your belly and creating the loving, open space for life. On the exhalations, visualize stress, defeating thoughts, frustration, etc. all leaving the body. Feel the muscles relax and get heavy with each exhalation. On the inhalations, invite the prana into every cell of your body. Feel your hands rise with your breath. Let the gentle rhythm of your breath take you deeper and deeper into relaxation. Set an intention related to your fertility journey. This can be as simple as "I intend to get pregnant and have a beautiful, healthy baby." It can also be something like, "I intend to be kind to myself in this process of trying to conceive." Continue this breathing until you feel calm, and the breath is smooth and even. Ideally, the inhale and exhale should be either equal in length, or the exhale should be a little longer. Allow there to be a bit of a pause at the end of the exhale, and the end of the inhale, before you start the next breath. This "space" is perhaps the most important part of the breath. Try at least 12 full inhales and exhales, but feel free to do more if your mind hasn't calmed after 12 breaths.

Why Do This?

This centering/calming breathing technique helps the body and mind relax. The deep, conscious breaths send signals to the nervous system that the muscles in the body can relax, and the mind can stop racing. Allowing the breath to expand the low belly helps us overcome cultural conditioning to hold in the abdomen, and helps to release tension in the pelvic area. Deep breathing is a wonderful way to begin your yoga practice. It can also be used on its own as a technique any time you need to relax.

POSES LYING ON YOUR BACK

2. KNEES TO CHEST

Setup

Now practice incorporating a simple movement with slow, conscious breathing. Bend your knees, and take your feet up off the floor. Place your hands on your knees.

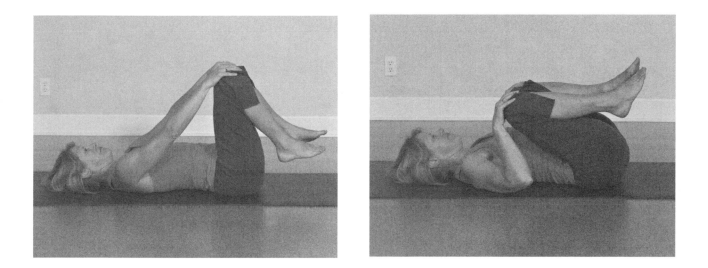

Movement

On an exhale, bring your knees gently toward your chest; don't hug them in, just gently draw them in. On your inhale, push the knees gently away as far as your arms can comfortably reach. The feet will remain off of the floor. Repeat the movement 5 to 8 more times. The focus should be mostly on the breath, rather than on the movement. Move slowly, using the whole exhale to bring the knees toward your chest, and the whole inhale to straighten your arms again.

Why Do This?

This simple movement allows you to get used to integrating the breath with movement. See if you can make your focus be on the breath, and just let the movement happen, with the breath leading the way. This is a very different approach than we use for most kinds of exercise—usually we are thinking about the activity or movement we need to do, and the breath just has to keep up. Now, we are trying to make it mostly about the breath, with the movement just following.

3. MOVING BRIDGE

Setup

Remain on your back with the knees bent and let the feet come down to the floor and rest hip-width apart (this is about 4–6 inches apart). The heels are not right next to the sitting bones; 6–8 inches away is about right. Let the palms of the hands rest on the floor on either side of your hips. Next, we will add a bit more movement, again coordinating the movement with the breath.

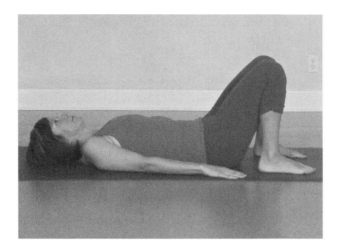

Movement

On an inhale, press both feet into the floor and lift the hips. At the same time, bring the arms up overhead until the hands touch the floor. On the exhale, slowly roll down, lowering the hips and the arms together. See if you can roll down one vertebra at a time. Notice if any part of the back wants to come down in a "chunk." If so, take extra time with this area. Use the whole inhale to come up, and the whole exhale to lower back down. Repeat for 5 to 8 full breaths. Pay attention to the feet, also. See if you can press all four corners of each foot into the floor.

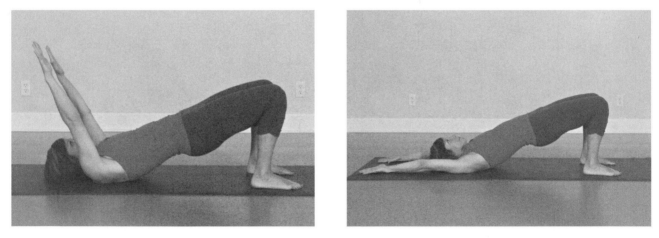

(**Modification:** If the shoulders are very tight, or if you have a shoulder injury, just leave the hands palms down and raise the hips only).

Why Do This?

Moving bridge pose opens the shoulders and chest, activates the feet, legs and buttocks, and opens the spine in two opposite directions. It also strengthens the abdominal organs. In addition, this pose provides more practice moving with the breath, where the breath is the main focus and the movement follows the breath.

4. **SUPPORTED BRIDGE

Setup

The Setup is the same as for **Moving Bridge**. Make sure you have a block close by.

Movement

On an inhale, press both feet and hands into the floor and lift the hips straight up. Place your block onto the floor just underneath your sacrum, which is the small triangular shaped bone at the base of the spine. You may have to move the block up or down to find the place that feels most comfortable. Place the block at the lowest height (widest side on the floor). Your arms can rest by your sides with the palms facing up, or you can place your hands on your belly. Allow your whole body to relax here. You may feel a release in the pelvis and low back. You can stay in this pose for up to 5 minutes. Take at least 10 breaths in the pose with the eyes closed. To come out of the pose, inhale and gently lift the hips enough to slide the block out to one side. Lower the hips and take a resting breath on your back. ** **Don't do this pose if you are in the main flow days of your period.**

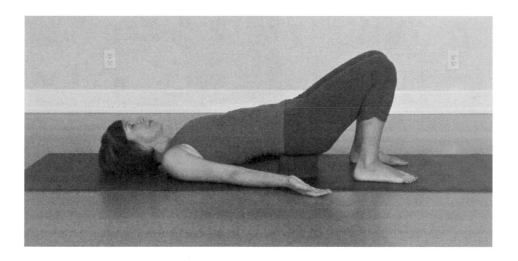

Why Do This?

Supported bridge releases tension in the pelvis and low back, and brings energy and vitality to the reproductive organs. It also helps to release tension in the neck and shoulders. Because of the slight downward angle, this pose helps to regulate the entire endocrine system. It is also very calming to the central nervous system.

5. SACRUM CIRCLES

Setup

Take the feet up off the floor, and put your hands on your knees.

Movement

Gently circle the knees one direction, keeping an even breath going with the circles. Try to have the movement follow the lead of the breath. After a few circles, pause and switch directions.

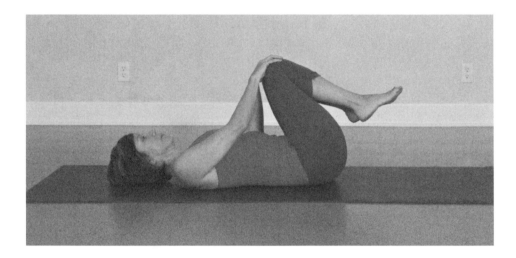

Why Do This?

This action massages the sacrum, (the flat bone at the lower end of the spine), and releases tension in the low back. In the yoga "map" of the body, the sacrum is part of the reproductive energy center, so keeping circulation and energy moving through this area is important. It is also another chance to practice adding a simple movement to the breath, while maintaining your focus on the breath.

6. OUTER HIP STRETCH (#4 POSE)

Setup

Find your strap. With your knees bent and feet on the floor, lift the right foot, and pass the strap around the right shin. Release the right foot back to the floor. Hold one end of the strap in each hand. Now, cross the left ankle inside the right knee. One end of the strap should come through the triangular space in the center between the two legs.

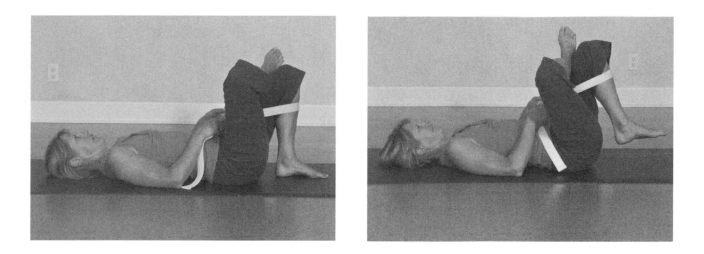

Movement

If you are already feeling a lot of stretch in the left outer hip or hamstring area, just keep the right foot on the floor and breathe. For more stretch, pull on the straps to draw the right knee gently toward the chest. Breathe with full, even breaths. Try 5–8 breaths here. Switch the legs and do the other side of the pose. Let the shoulders relax as much as possible while holding the strap. Relax the face muscles, too. See how many muscles in the body you can relax while allowing the outer hip rotators to stretch. (**Modification:** If you have knee injuries, don't take the strap around the shin. Instead, pass the strap under the knee).

Why Do This?

We are stretching the rotator muscles in the outer hips, which are a group of short, but powerful muscles that are tight on many people. This is because just about everything we do on a regular basis tightens them—including walking, sitting, and many other common, everyday activities. Releasing tension in these muscles also releases tension in the pelvic area, and allows energy and blood flow to move more easily through this area. This stretch also helps alleviate low back problems.

7. HAPPY BABY POSE

Setup

With your knees bent and feet on the floor, lift your feet, one at a time, so that the soles of your feet are up toward the ceiling. Keep the knees bent. If you are flexible enough, you can take the hands to the outer or inner edges of the feet. However, if your shoulders and sacrum are off the floor when you do this, it would be better to take a strap around each foot, and hold both ends of each strap, instead of holding the feet.

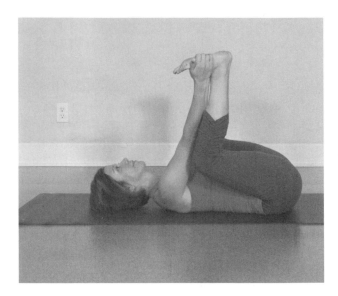

Movement

Holding either the straps or the feet, start to draw the knees down toward the armpits. Keep the soles of the feet up toward the ceiling, and the sacrum down toward the floor.

Why Do This?

This pose is a great hip opener, and helps to increase the blood flow into the pelvic area.

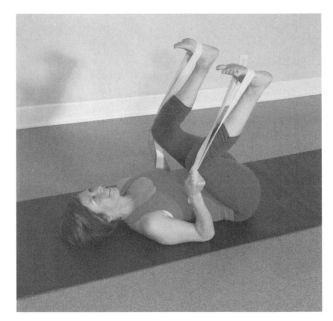

8. PELVIC TILTS

Setup

Setup is the same as for **Moving Bridge**.

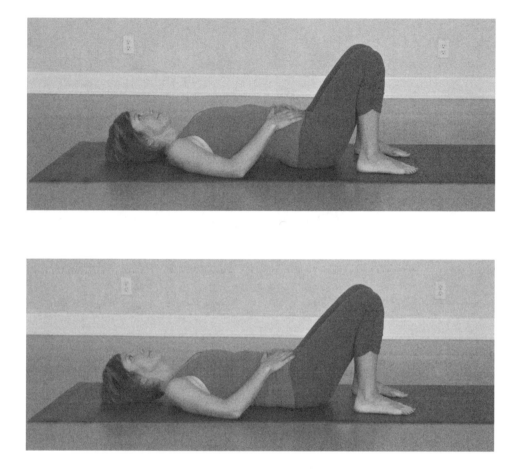

Movement

With an exhale, *gently* press the low back down into the floor. On the inhale release and let the low back come up again. Repeat for 5 to 8 breaths.

Why Do This?

While there are versions of this which are used for core strengthening, that is not our purpose here. We are using this pose to create a gentle rocking of the pelvis. This encourages blood and energy flow, and releases tension and stagnation in the pelvis. For this purpose, press the low back down *gently*, trying not to engage the abdominal muscles any more than necessary to get the action to happen.

9. BENT KNEE TWIST (SECOND HALF VERSION)

Setup

With your knees bent and feet on the floor, take the feet to the outer edges of your yoga mat. The feet will be about two feet apart. Now, take the arms out to the sides like a "T," with your palms facing up.

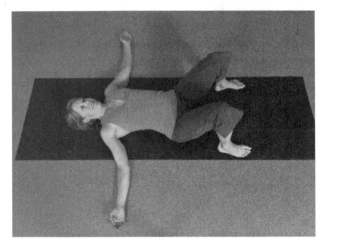 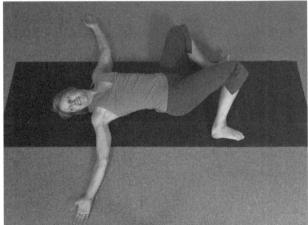

Movement

Lift the hips and shift them slightly toward the left. Then allow the knees to drop over toward the right, keeping the feet touching the mat. You don't need to keep the entire sole of the foot on the floor; it can be the edge of the foot that is still touching the floor. Turn the head to look back toward the left palm. Take several slow, even breaths. On an inhale, bring the knees back to center, and do the twist to the second side.

Why Do This?

Twists are cleansing and rejuvenating for the organs (such as the uterus and intestines) and glands (such as the ovaries) in the abdominal area. Twists have a calming effect on the central nervous system.

10. COMING UP

Setup

Bend your knees and roll onto your right side, with both knees bent. Take a breath or two on your right side.

Movement

Use both hands to gently press yourself back up to a seated position.

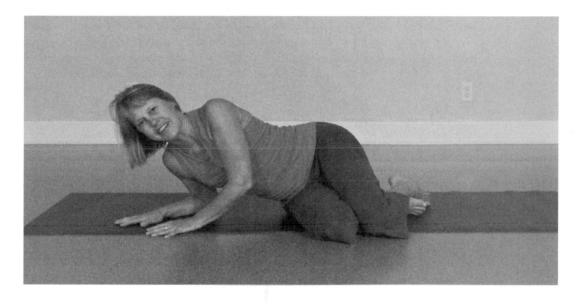

Why Do This?

Rolling to the side and pressing the floor inhibits tension in the neck and lower back. Rolling to the right side keeps the heart on top, so that you don't compress the heart (which is located on the left side). It also keeps the pulse regular, and frees up the breath through the left nostril, which promotes relaxation.

❁ POSES ON HANDS AND KNEES

11. CAT-COW

Setup

Come onto your hands and knees with your wrists underneath your shoulders and your knees underneath your hips. Your knees should be 4–6 inches apart. Spread the fingers wide apart from each other. If this position bothers your knees, you can try folding a blanket and placing it underneath your knees for extra padding.

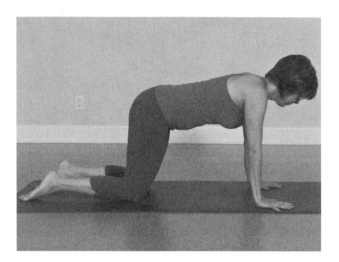

Movement

On an inhale, tilt your tailbone up and arch your back. Look forward and draw the shoulders back away from the ears. Keep your core engaged as you arch the back. On an exhale, tilt your tailbone down toward the floor and round your spine. Press the shoulder blades up toward the ceiling. Let your head and neck feel heavy. Repeat at least 5 times, initiating each movement at the tailbone. Allow the movement to follow the breath.

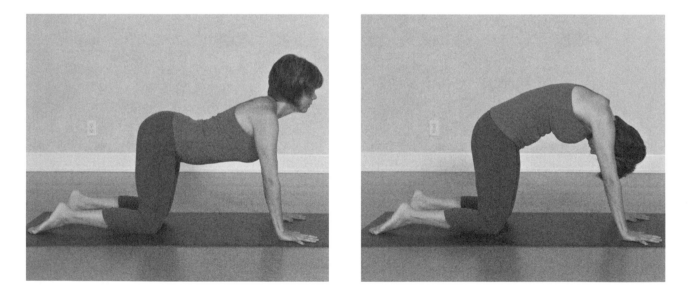

Why Do This?

Cat-cow warms up all of the muscles in the back and allows tension in the neck and shoulders to release. It also opens the major energy channels in the front and back of the body. The pelvic movements bring blood flow and energy through the pelvis.

12. CAT-COW CIRCLES

Setup

Setup is the same as for Cat-Cow.

Movement

Circle the hips and ribcage around to the right, bending the elbows as much as you need to. This is a very free-form movement, so just do what feels good to your body. You may get some forward-and-back movement as well as the circling. Don't forget to breathe while performing these circles. After a few breaths, switch directions.

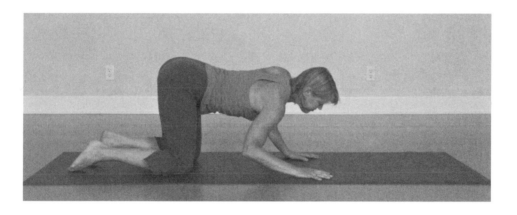

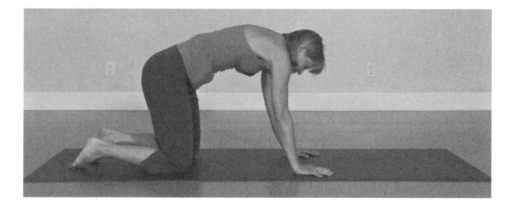

Why Do This?

The circling motion releases tension in the pelvis, ribcage and shoulders. We are taking the torso through a range of motion that most of us don't experience in our regular daily lives, so it encourages us to release physical and emotional patterns where we may be "stuck."

13.   PRAYER POSE (CHILD'S POSE)

Setup

From the hands and knees position, take the knees wide apart and sit the hips back onto the heels. Keep the toes together. Bring the forehead to the floor, and reach the arms forward with the palms facing down. If it isn't comfortable to bring the forehead all the way to the floor, you can stack the hands one on top of each other, and rest the forehead on the hands, or rest the forehead on a block or a folded blanket. Let the toes release.

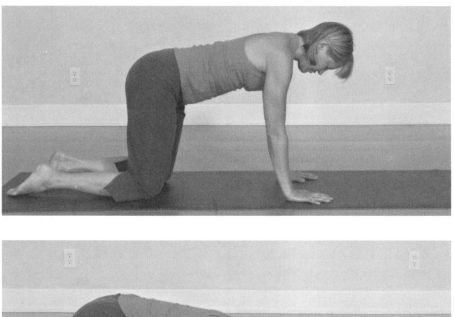

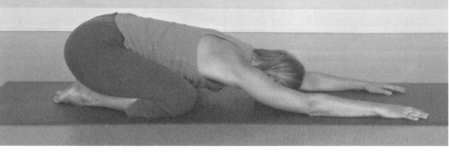

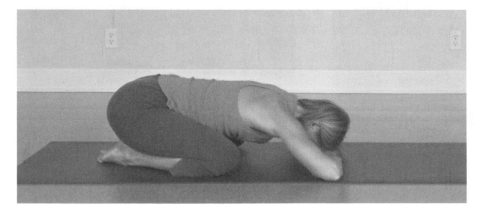

Movement

Prayer pose is a resting pose, so in the standard version of prayer pose, you are resting here, rather than moving. To come up from prayer pose, just walk the hands back in toward the body, and come up slowly.

Variations

Try a couple of variations of prayer pose which include some movement: *Variation 1)* In prayer pose, gently and slowly move the hips side to side, stretching out each side of the low back. *Variation 2)* On an exhale, creep the hands over to the right side of the mat, until you get a stretch in the left side of the body. You can optionally turn the head and look toward the right, to get some stretch into the neck. Take a few breaths here. On an inhale, creep the hands back to center, and on the next exhale, repeat the pose on the left side.

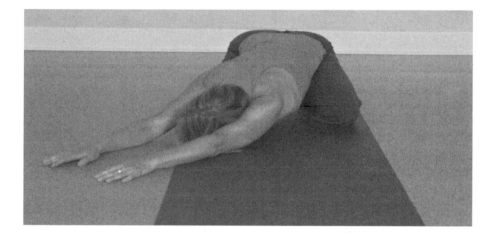

Why Do This?

Prayer pose is known for its calming effect, which is partly due to resting the forehead down. It also stretches and relaxes the low back and opens the shoulders.

14. DOWNWARD FACING DOG

Setup

From the hands and knees position, take an inhale and engage the muscles of the arms. Relax the space between your shoulder blades.

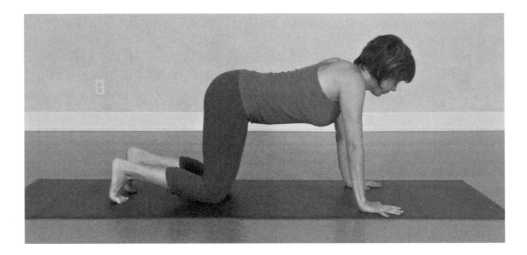

Movement

Exhale, curl your toes under and lift your knees off of the floor. Lift the hips, and draw the low belly up and back. Press strongly through the hands, and draw energy from the hands up the arms. Take a peek back at your feet and be sure they are "sitting-bones-width" distance apart (about 4–6 inches apart) and parallel. Keep the undersides of the arms lifting away from the floor. Your heels may or may not touch the floor. If you feel a lot of stretch in your hamstrings, bend the knees slightly, allowing the back to lengthen. Stay here for a few breaths feeling the whole body stretch and lengthen. **Don't stay in this pose for an extended length of time if you are on the main flow days of your period.**

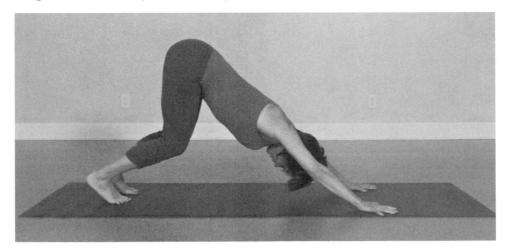

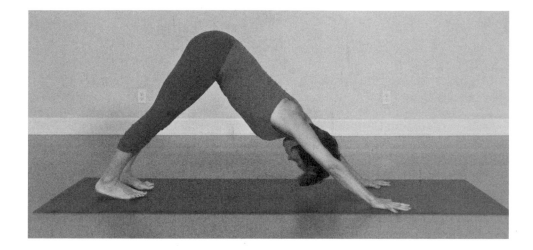

Why Do This?

Downward dog is a full body stretch that is good for the whole body. It is also an inversion which is beneficial for the circulatory system as well as for the endocrine system. It tones the abdominal muscles, opens the shoulders, and can help regulate problems with the menstrual cycle. However, you should not do this pose for an extended period of time during the main flow days of your period. From a fertility perspective, it opens the energy channel between the heart and the uterus. In the Chinese medicine tradition, opening this energy channel is one of the keys to conception.

15. PRAYER POSE VARIATION

Setup

Come into **Prayer Pose**. Move hips gently side-to-side in prayer pose to release low back.

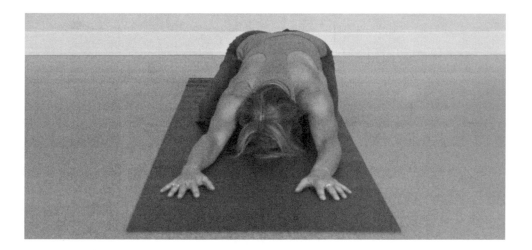

16. KNEE-DOWN LUNGE

Setup

From prayer pose, walk your hands back in toward your body, raising your torso.

Movement

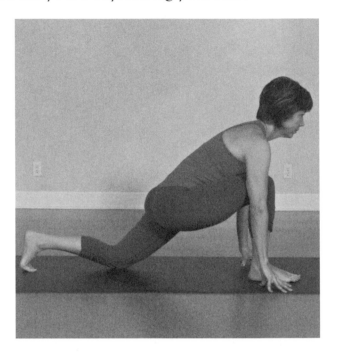

Step your right foot forward between your hands and curl your back toes under so you are pressing the ball of the left foot into the floor. Squeeze the legs in towards an imaginary midline down the center of your body. The hands can remain on the floor, on either side of the front foot, or you can and place both hands on your right thigh. Stay here or reach your arms over your head. Take five full breaths in this pose. Retrace your steps carefully until you are back to a tabletop position on your hands and knees. Repeat steps on the left side. After the second side, step the right foot forward and come up to a standing position at the front of your mat.

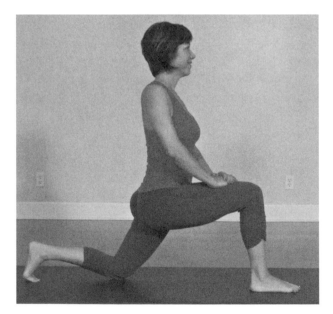

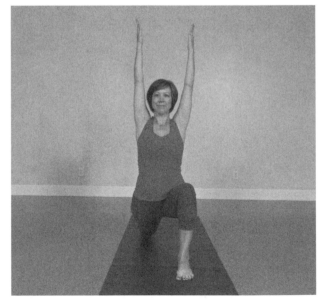

Why Do This?

This pose tones the abdominal organs including the reproductive organs. It opens the quadriceps, which allows more circulation and energy to flow into the pelvic area.

✦ STANDING POSES

17. MOUNTAIN POSE

Setup

Stand with your feet hip-width apart (about 4–6 inches) and parallel. Allow the arms to rest gently by your sides.

Movement

Make sure your feet are not turned out or in. Try to balance the weight evenly on the front and backs of the feet and on the inner and outer edges of the feet. Notice if your knees are collapsing in toward each other and bring the knees over the ankles. Also be sure not to hyperextend your knee joints. Ideally your pelvis will be in a neutral position. Be sure that your shoulders are over your hips and your neck and chin are not jutting out. Lengthen the crown of your head toward the sky and take 5 to 8 breaths.

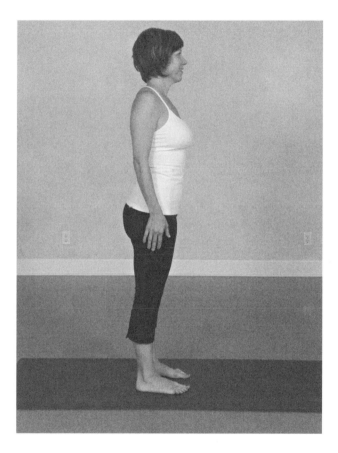

Why Do This?

Mountain pose can be practiced anywhere. It helps you develop body awareness and good posture for breathing. It also tones the abdominal organs.

18. TREE POSE

Setup

Begin by standing in Mountain Pose.

Movement

Bring the weight into your left foot and leg and bend your right knee and place it on your left ankle, calf or thigh. Bring your palms together in front of your heart, or extend your arms over your head in a V shape. Find a point to focus your eyes on, either straight in front of you, or on the floor ahead of you. This helps with balance. Stay here for 5 to 8 breaths. Retrace your steps slowly to release the pose and repeat on the opposite side.

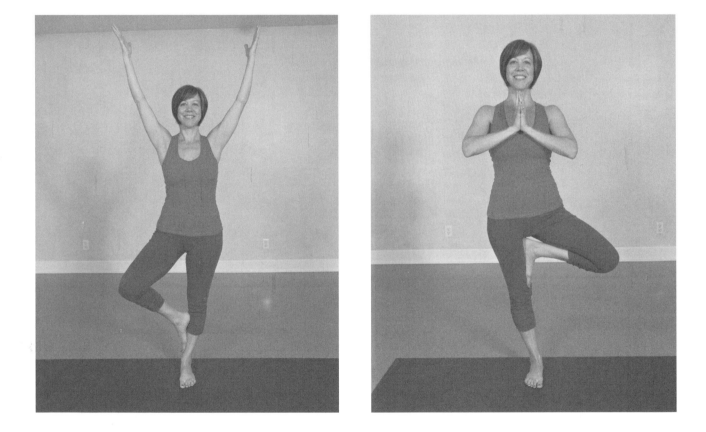

Why Do This?

This pose helps opens the hips and develops balance, focus, strength and patience. It is a great pose for working on the concept of being present during your yoga practice. If your mind wanders in this pose, you usually get instant feedback!

19. SIDE ANGLE POSE

Setup

Facing the long side of your mat, step your feet about 3 ½ to 4 feet apart. Turn your right foot out 90 degrees so that the outer edge of your foot aligns with the side of your mat. Keep your left foot pointing straight ahead or turn it in slightly.

Movement

Bend your right knee towards 90 degrees keeping your knee over your ankle. Lean to the right and place your right forearm just above your knee. Place your left hand on your waist and turn your torso toward the sky. Stay here or extend your left arm over your head, keeping the bicep over the ear with the palm facing down. Anchor this forward movement by firmly pressing the outer edge of the back foot into the floor. Take 4–5 breaths. To come up, press down through the feet and legs and bring your torso back up to vertical on an inhale. Pivot the feet so the left foot turns out to 90 degrees and the right foot points straight ahead or turns in slightly. Repeat steps above on the left side.

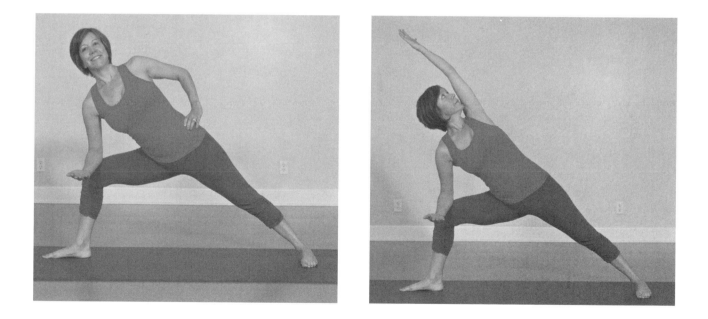

Why Do This?

Side angle pose tones the pelvic organs and can also help with menstrual problems. It creates length and space in the torso, nourishing the organs and glands.

20. SQUAT POSE AND VARIATIONS

Setup

Stand with feet wider than hip-width apart, approximately 12 inches to start. The closer your feet are together, the more difficult squat pose is.

Movement

Bend the knees and lower the sitting bones toward the floor, keeping the back long and the crown of the head up toward the ceiling. The heels should be down on the floor in squat pose. If they don't come to the floor, try taking the feet wider apart or turning the feet out slightly (turning the feet out increases the strain on the knees, though!). If the heels are still off the floor, try one of the variations below. Now, take the palms of the hands together, and press the elbows toward the inner knees to help open the groin and hips.

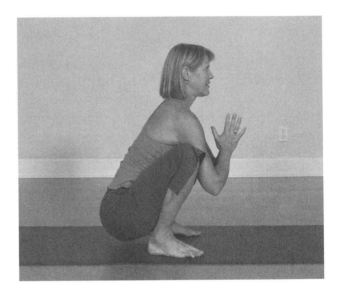

Why Do This?

Squat pose opens the groin, the hips and the pelvic floor, and lengthens the spine. It also strengthens the quadriceps muscles along the front of the legs. You may also feel a nice stretch in the low back.

Don't do this pose if you have knee injuries, as squat pose can stress the knee joint. In this case, you can choose the "squat on a block" variation below, or skip squat altogether.

Variations on Squat Pose

If you are not able to get your heels to the floor in squat pose, try one of these options.

1. **Support your heels** on a rolled blanket or yoga mat.

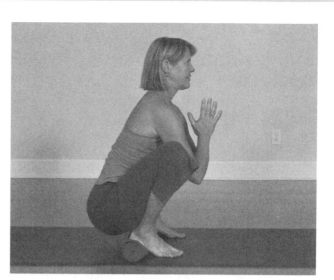

2. **Place your back against a wall.** With feet 12 inches apart, and about 8–10 inches away from the wall, slide down the wall to squat pose. If your heels are not on the ground, adjust the distance your feet are from the wall, so that your heels are down. Allow as much of the spine as possible to rest back against the wall.

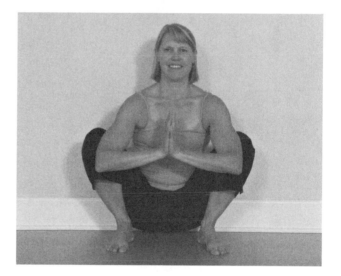

3. **Use a block** underneath the buttocks to support you in squat pose.

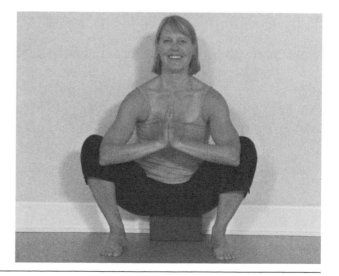

SEATED POSES

21. "CHICKEN WING" SHOULDER STRETCH

Setup

Sit in a comfortable seated, cross-legged position. You may want to sit up on one or two folded blankets if your hips, knees or low back are uncomfortable when sitting on the mat without support. Make sure you are sitting straight down on your sitting bones, not leaning forward or rounding the low back. Take your hands onto your shoulders with the fingers forward, thumbs behind, elbows out to the sides.

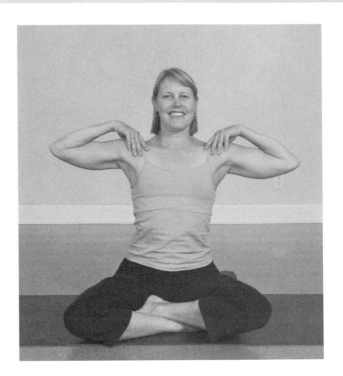

Movement

Inhale and raise the elbows up toward the ceiling. Shrug the shoulders slightly and lengthen the sides of the body. Exhale audibly, through the mouth, lowering the elbows all the way back down next to your rib cage. Repeat 4–6 times.

Why Do This?

This pose reduces shoulder tension, and opens and lengthens the sides of the body, improving circulation and energy flow. Audible exhales with the mouth open help clear energy blockages in the throat center.

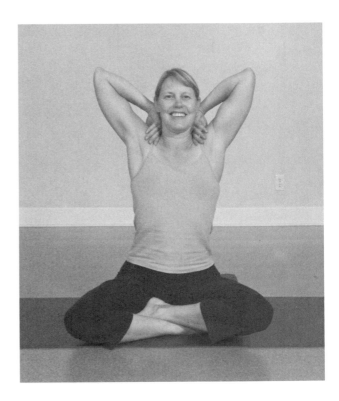

22. SEATED WIDE-LEG STRADDLE

Setup

Sit on a mat or a blanket with the legs apart, feet flexed, toes and knees facing straight up. You don't need to take your legs as wide apart as you can, just a comfortable distance apart. Be sure there is a natural curve in the low back. If your back is rounding, add another blanket underneath you.

Movement

Place your hands on the floor behind you. On an inhale, lengthen your spine and expand your chest while pressing the backs of the legs down into the floor. You can stay here for 5–8 breaths or you can take the hands in front of you, and begin to walk the hands forward, bringing the chest toward the floor. Only go as far forward as your spine allows. You will know you have gone too far if your back begins to round.

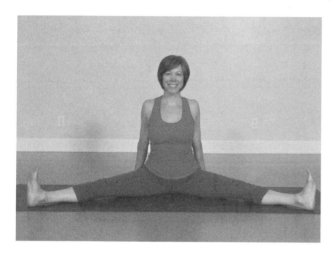
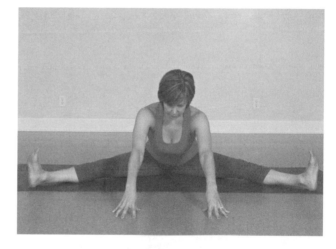

Variation

Turn your chest toward your right leg and stretch toward that leg for 3–5 breaths. You may want to use a strap around the right foot in this pose. Repeat on left side.

Why Do This?

This pose massages the reproductive organs and stimulates the ovaries. It can also help regulate menstrual flow. As with all forward bending poses, this is a calming pose.

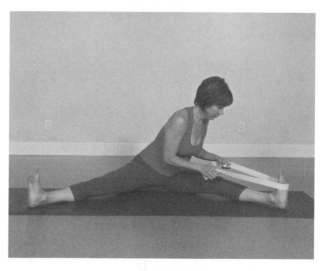

23. COBBLER POSE

Setup

Begin by sitting on your mat, or raise the hips by sitting on a folded blanket. Take the soles of the feet together, gently allowing the knees to open toward the floor.

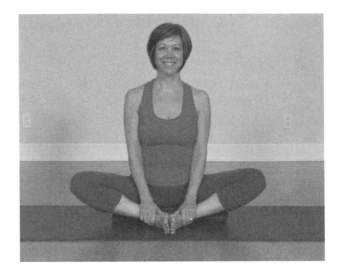

Movement

Place your hands behind your hips on the floor in back of you. On an inhale, lengthen your spine and expand your chest while allowing the knees to open gently down toward the floor. On an exhale, roll your shoulders down and back. You can stay here for 5–8 breaths, or you can take your hands to your feet, bringing the chest down towards the floor. Only go as far forward as your spine allows. You will know you have gone too far if your back begins to round.

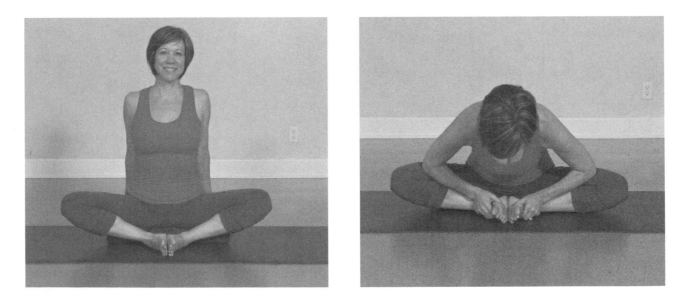

Why Do This?

This pose relaxes the pelvic area, and improves energy flow and blood circulation in the pelvis.

⚜ RELAXATION POSES

24. **LEGS UP THE WALL POSE (WITH VARIATIONS)

Setup

Do this pose at a clear space of wall, where you have room to take your legs straight up the wall without bumping into anything. Before you start, put on warm clothes and socks, and have a blanket handy which you can pull over yourself once you get into the pose. Place your yoga mat lengthwise to the wall.

Movement

Start by sitting sideways at the wall, with your right hip just next to the wall and your knees bent. Place your left hand on the floor next to your left hip, and your right hand on the floor behind you. Lean back, and take some weight onto your hands. You might even come down onto your elbows. Next, you will need to swing your legs up the wall, so that your sitting bones end up fairly close to the wall. The actual "best" distance from the wall depends partly on your hamstring flexibility. Find a place where your hamstrings are not unhappy when your legs are up the wall. (If your hamstrings are tight, it may help to place a folded blanket on the mat next to the wall, and sit on the blanket to start. Or, take the sitting bones a little further from the wall.) **Don't do this if you are on the main flow days of your period.**

Variations

You can keep the legs a few inches apart on the wall, or try varying the leg position by taking them wider apart, or taking the soles of the feet together like Cobbler Pose. The hands can rest on the low belly, or on either side of you about 12 inches away from the body, with the palms facing up toward the ceiling.

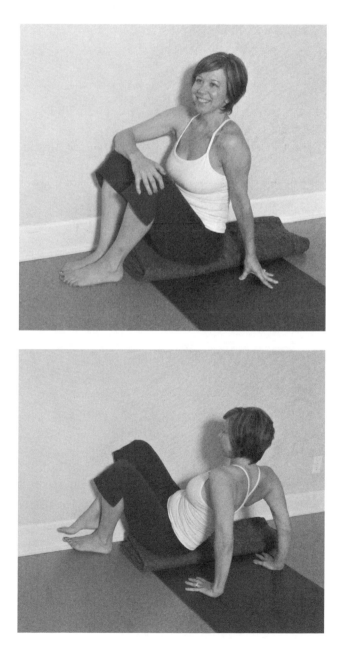

This is a resting pose, so make yourself as comfortable as possible. Take care not to get chilled as you are resting. This pose may take a few practice tries, and may feel awkward at first. This is a very important fertility pose—so don't give up. When you get ready to come out of the pose, draw the knees into the chest and roll onto your right side with your knees bent. Rest for a few breaths before using both hands to press up to a seated position.

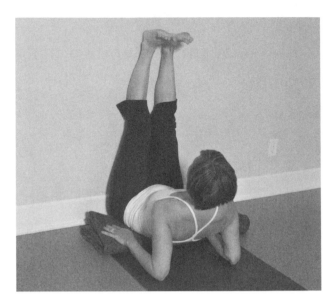

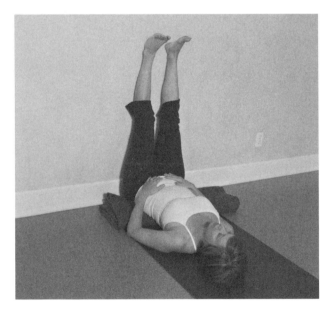

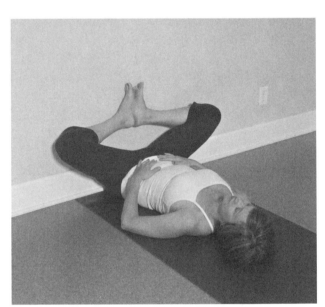

Why Do This?

You may feel like you are doing nothing once you get into the pose, but don't be fooled. This pose is one of the most powerful fertility-supporting yoga poses that you can practice. The abdominal organs are nourished and revitalized when the blood from the feet and legs pools in the low belly. Toxins are removed from the bloodstream, as the blood flows into the lymph glands in the groin. The central nervous system is calmed and the endocrine system is regulated. It is a great pose to do just before bedtime, as it promotes restful sleep. This pose should be done daily for at least 5 minutes, during every part of the cycle except when you are menstruating. You may want to choose one of the visualizations from Chapter 7 to do while you are in this pose.

25. CORPSE POSE

Setup

Lie on your back with your feet and legs relaxed and apart. Allow your arms to rest by your sides a few inches away from your body with your palms facing up. If you have tension or pain in your lower back, place a rolled up blanket or bolster underneath your knees. For added relaxation, place an eye pillow over your eyes.

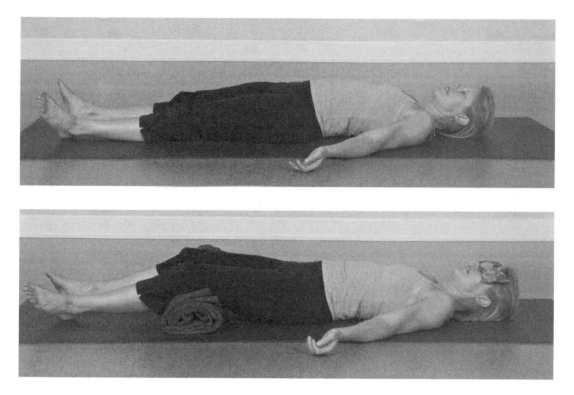

Movement

Feel the support of the floor beneath you, and with each exhale allow your body to feel heavy and relaxed. There is no effort needed here. Tuck your chin ever so slightly toward your chest so the back of the neck is long. Relax and open your palms toward the sky, ready to receive the gifts of your practice. If your mind begins to wander, acknowledge that tendency and let the thoughts come and go with each breath. Stay in this pose for 5–7 minutes or even longer if you have time.

Why Do This?

Corpse pose allows all of the benefits of your practice to integrate into your body, mind and spirit. It can help relieve stress and mild depression, and lower blood pressure. Corpse pose can help with insomnia, fatigue and headaches. It also encourages the mind to rest, as the body sinks into a state of deep relaxation.

✿ YOGA FOR FERTILITY: SECOND HALF INTERMEDIATE ROUTINE

The following sequence can be done if you are a more experienced yoga practitioner, or if you have built up your confidence with the basic routine. These poses are ideal for the second half of your cycle after ovulation has occurred. We are focusing on bringing energy and blood flow to the uterus so the lining will continue to thicken to support implantation. These poses are all safe if you become pregnant and can be performed up until the third month of pregnancy. You can also go to Chapter 6 for a Prenatal Yoga Sequence that can be used throughout your first trimester.

SUMMARY FLOW OF SECOND HALF INTERMEDIATE ROUTINE

Note: A double asterisk (**) means you should not practice this pose during the main flow days of your period.

1. **Centering/Calming Breath (Belly Breath)**

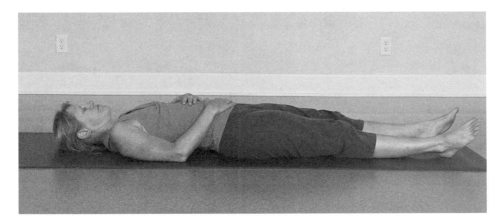

2. **Moving Bridge**

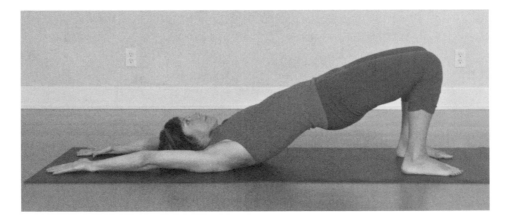

3. **Sacrum Circles**

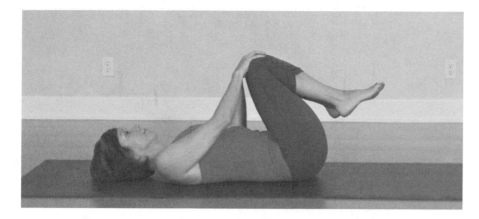

4. **Happy Baby Pose**

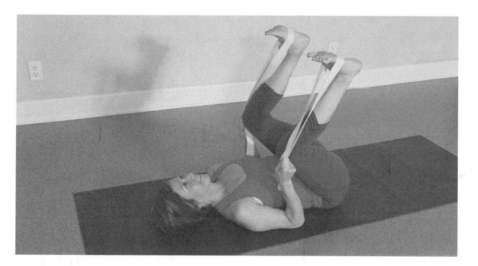

5. **Cat-Cow**

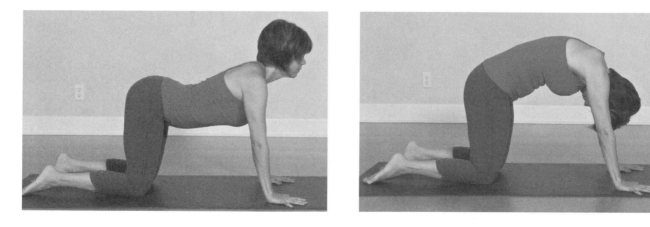

6. Cat-Cow Circles

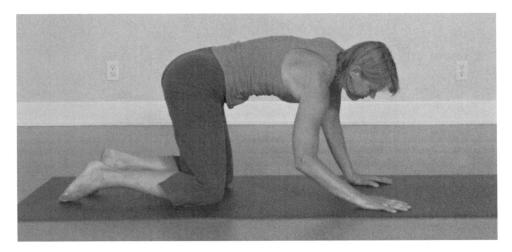

7. Downward Facing Dog

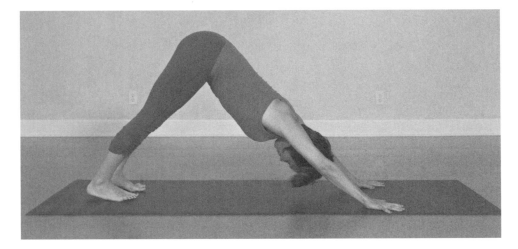

8. Prayer Pose (Child's Pose)

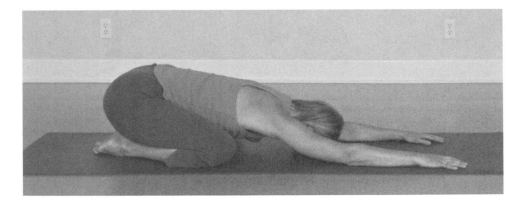

9. Pigeon Pose

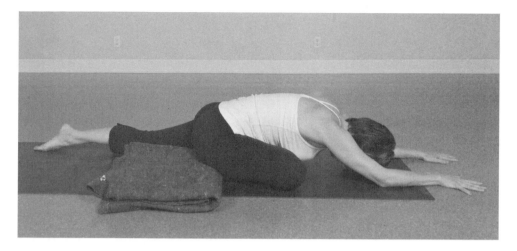

10. Side Angle Pose

11. Triangle Pose

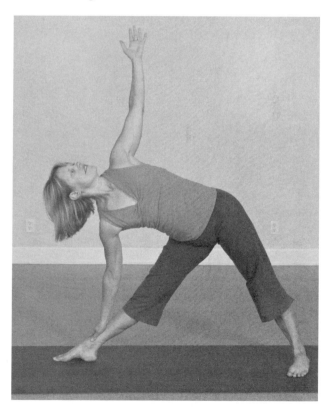

12. Half-Moon Balance Pose

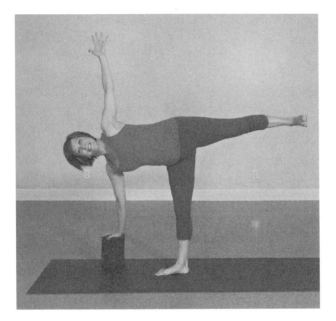

13. Squat Pose

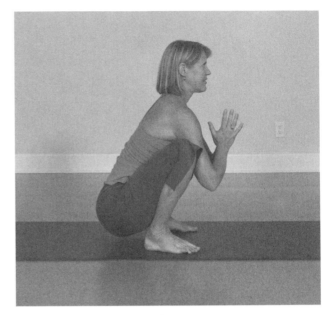

14. Wide standing Forward Bend with Immune Booster

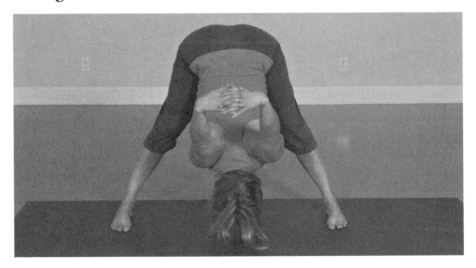

15. **Forward Bend over One Leg**

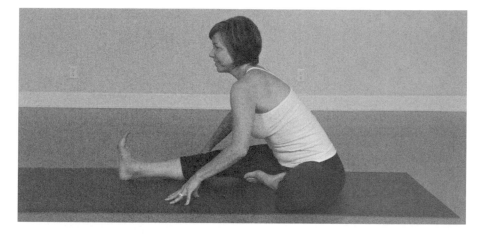

16. **Cobbler Pose with Heart Opener**

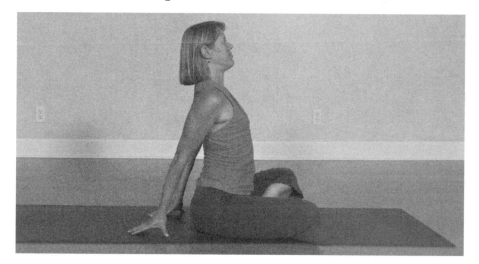

17. **Seated Wide-Leg Straddle**

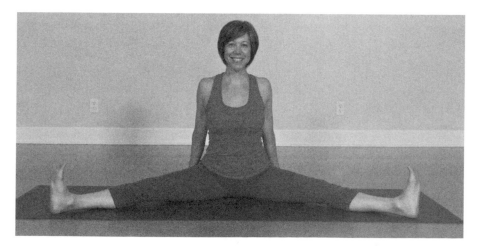

18. Pelvic Tilts

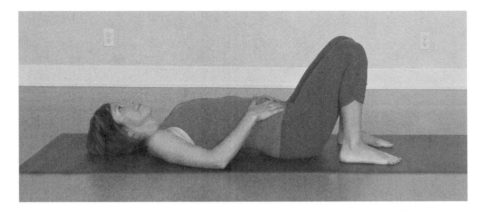

19. **Bridge Pose

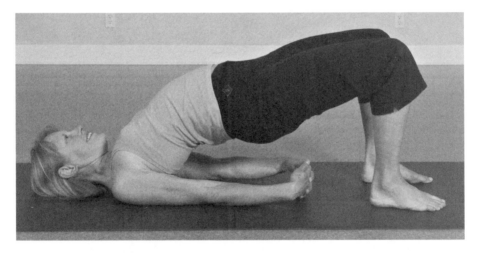

20. Bent Knee Twist (Second Half Version)

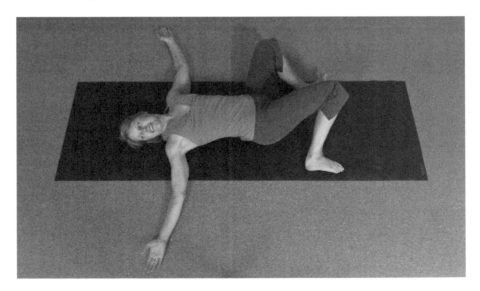

21. ****Legs up the Wall Pose**

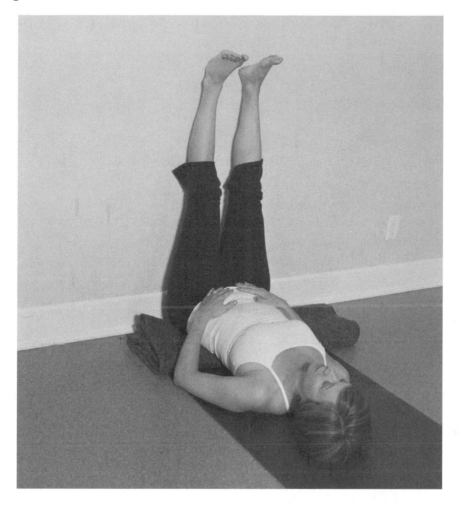

22. **Corpse Pose**

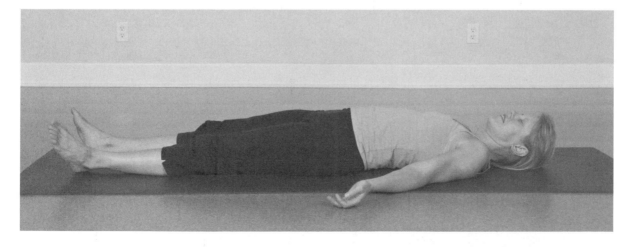

✿ POSE DESCRIPTIONS FOR SECOND HALF INTERMEDIATE ROUTINE

Note: A double asterisk (**) means you should not practice this pose during the main flow days of your period.

I. CENTERING/CALMING BREATH (BELLY BREATH)

Setup

This breath can be performed either seated or lying down. Lie on your back on your mat with your legs straight, or bend the knees if that is more comfortable for your low back. Another option is to sit in a chair with a solid seat that will allow you to sit with a long spine. Let your body relax and place your hands on your low belly.

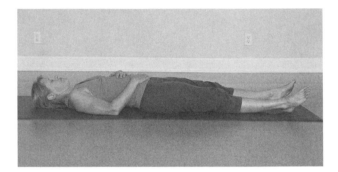

Movement

Breathe fully and deeply into your abdominal region, visualizing the prana (life force energy) filling your belly and creating the loving, open space for life. On the exhalations, visualize stress, defeating thoughts, frustration, etc. all leaving the body. Feel the muscles relax and get heavy with each exhalation. On the inhalations, invite the prana into every cell of your body. Feel your hands rise with your breath. Let the gentle rhythm of your breath take you deeper and deeper into relaxation. Set an intention related to your fertility journey. This can be as simple as "I intend to get pregnant and have a beautiful, healthy baby." It can also be something like, "I intend to be kind to myself in this process of trying to conceive." Continue this breathing until you feel calm, and the breath is smooth and even. Ideally, the inhale and exhale should be either equal in length, or the exhale should be a little longer. Allow there to be a bit of a pause at the end of the exhale, and the end of the inhale, before you start the next breath. This "space" is perhaps the most important part of the breath. Try at least 12 full inhales and exhales, but feel free to do more if your mind hasn't calmed after 12 breaths.

Why Do This?

This centering/calming breathing technique helps the body and mind relax. The deep, conscious breaths send signals to the nervous system that the muscles in the body can relax, and the mind can stop racing. Allowing the breath to expand the low belly helps us overcome cultural conditioning to hold in the abdomen, and helps to release tension in the pelvic area. Deep breathing is a wonderful way to begin your yoga practice. It can also be used on its own as a technique any time you need to relax.

✺ POSES LYING ON YOUR BACK

2. MOVING BRIDGE

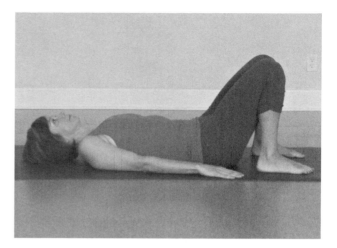

Setup

Lie on your back with your knees bent and feet on the floor hip-width apart (about 4 to 6 inches). Place the heels are not right next to the sitting bones; 6–8 inches away is about right. Let the palms of the hands rest on the floor on either side of your hips.

Movement

On an inhale, press all four corners of the feet into the floor and lift the hips. At the same time, bring the arms up overhead until the hands touch the floor.

On the exhale, slowly roll down, lowering the hips and the arms together. See if you can roll down one vertebra at a time. Notice if any part of the back wants to come down in a "chunk." If so, take extra time with this area. Use the whole inhale to raise up, and the whole exhale to lower back down. Repeat for 5 to 8 full breaths.

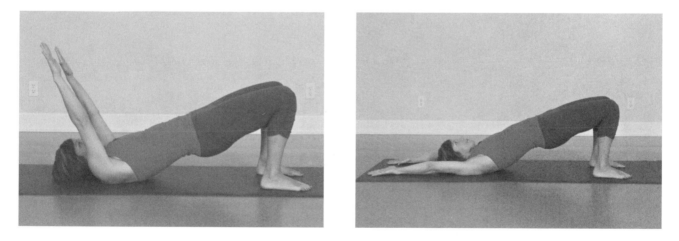

(*Modification:* if the shoulders are very tight, or if you have a shoulder injury, just leave the hands palms down on the floor and raise the hips only).

Why Do This?

Moving bridge pose opens the shoulders and chest, activates the feet, legs and buttocks, and opens the spine in two opposite directions. It also strengthens the abdominal organs. This pose provides more practice moving with the breath, where the breath is the main focus and the movement follows the breath.

3. SACRUM CIRCLES

Setup

Remain on your back as you bend the knees and take the feet up off the floor.

Movement

Place the hands on the knees and gently circle the knees one direction, keeping a nice even breath going with the circles. Try to make this mostly about the breath, with the movement just following the lead of the breath. After a few circles, pause and switch directions.

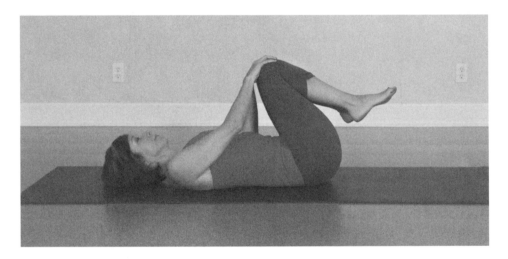

Why Do This?

This action massages the sacrum, (the flat bone at the lower end of the spine), and releases tension in the low back. In the yoga "map" of the body, the sacrum is part of the reproductive energy center, so keeping circulation and energy moving through this area is important. It is also another chance to practice adding a simple movement to the breath, while maintaining your focus on the breath.

4. HAPPY BABY POSE

Setup

With your knees bent and feet on the floor, lift your feet, one at a time, so that the soles of your feet are up toward the ceiling. Keep the knees bent. If you are flexible enough, you can take the hands to the outer or inner edges of the feet. However, if your shoulders and sacrum are off the floor when you do this, it would be better to take a strap around each foot, and hold both ends of each strap, instead of holding the foot.

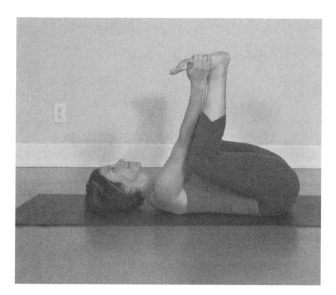

Movement

Now, holding either the straps or the feet, start to draw the knees down toward the armpits. Keep the soles of the feet up toward the ceiling, and the sacrum down toward the floor.

Why Do This?

This pose is a great hip opener, and helps to increase the blood flow into the pelvic area.

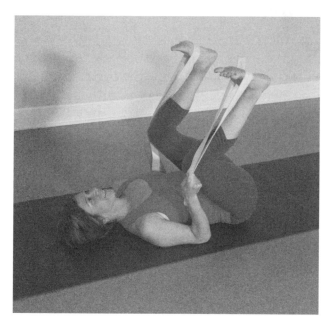

✦ POSES ON HANDS AND KNEES

5. CAT-COW

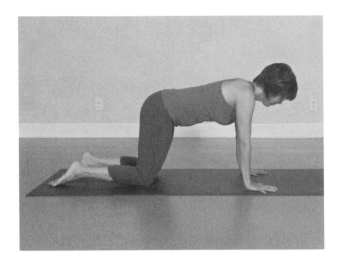

Setup

Come onto your hands and knees with your wrists underneath your shoulders and your knees underneath your hips. Spread the fingers wide apart from each other. Your knees should be 4–6 inches apart from each other. If this position bothers your knees, you can try folding a blanket and placing it underneath your knees for extra padding.

Movement

On an inhale, tilt your tailbone up and arch your back. Look forward and draw the shoulders back away from the ears. Keep your core engaged as you arch the back. On an exhale, tilt your tailbone down toward the floor and round your spine. Press the shoulder blades up toward the ceiling. Let your head and neck feel heavy. Repeat 5–8 times, initiating each movement at the tailbone. Allow the movement to follow the breath.

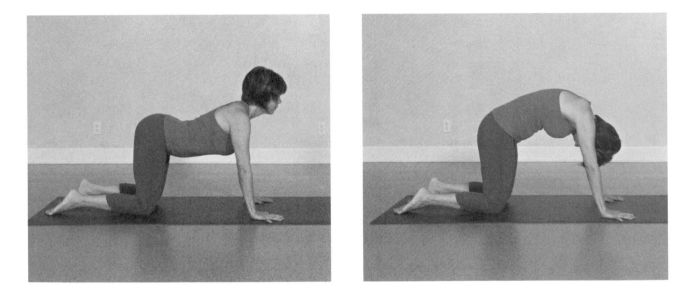

Why Do This?

Cat-cow warms up all of the muscles in the back and allows tension in the neck and shoulders to release. It also opens the major energy channels in the front and back of the body. The pelvic movements bring blood flow and energy through the pelvis.

6. CAT-COW CIRCLES

Setup

Setup is the same as for Cat-Cow.

Movement

Circle the hips and ribcage around to the right, bending the elbows as much as you need to. This is a very free-form movement, so just do what feels good to your body. You may get some forward-and-back movement as well as the circling. Don't forget to breathe while performing these circles. After a few breaths, switch directions.

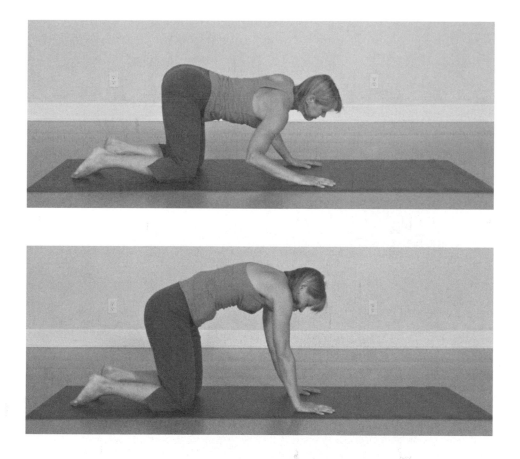

Why Do This?

The circling motion releases tension in the pelvis, ribcage and shoulders. We are taking the torso through a range of motion that most of us don't experience in our regular daily lives, so it encourages us to release physical and emotional patterns where we may be "stuck."

7. DOWNWARD FACING DOG

Setup

From the hands and knees position, take an inhale and engage the muscles of the arms. Relax the space between your shoulder blades.

Movement

Exhale, curl your toes under and lift your knees off of the floor. Lift the hips, and draw the low belly up and back. Press strongly through the hands, and draw energy from the hands up the arms. Take a peek back at your feet and be sure they are "sitting-bones-width" distance apart (about 4–6 inches apart) and parallel. Keep the undersides of the arms lifting away from the floor. Your heels may or may not touch the floor. If you feel a lot of stretch in your hamstrings, bend the knees slightly, allowing the back to lengthen. Stay here for three to five breaths, feeling the whole body stretch and lengthen. **Do not do this pose for an extended length of time during the main flow days of your period.**

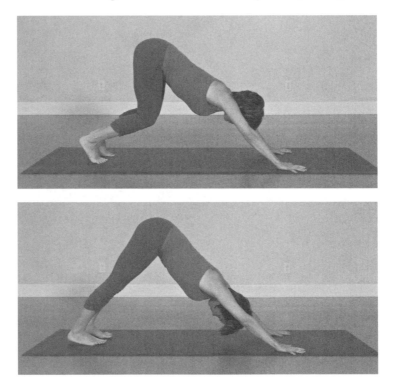

Why Do This?

Downward facing dog is a full body stretch that is good for the whole body. It is also an inversion which is beneficial for the circulatory system as well as for the endocrine system. It tones the abdominal muscles and can help relieve menstrual problems. However, you should not do this pose for an extended length of time during the main flow days of your period.

8. PRAYER POSE (CHILD'S POSE)

Setup

From the hands and knees position, take the knees wide apart and sit the hips back onto the heels. Keep the toes together. Bring the forehead to the floor, and reach the arms forward with the palms facing down. Let the toes release.

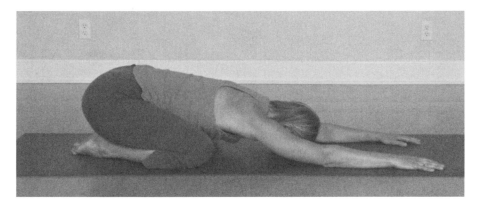

Movement

Prayer pose is a resting pose, so in the standard version of prayer pose, you are resting here, rather than moving. To come up from prayer pose, just walk the hands back in toward the body, and come up slowly.

Variation (Child's Pose)

In prayer pose, reach the arms back along the outside of the calves, rather than reaching forward.

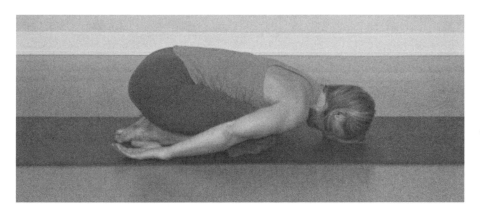

Why Do This?

Prayer pose is a resting pose that is known for its calming effect. It also stretches and relaxes the low back.

9. PIGEON POSE

Setup

Begin on your hands and knees in a table-top position.

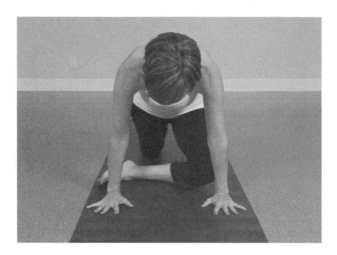

Movement

Slide your left knee toward your left hand, bringing the left foot in front of the right hip. Your left knee should be on the floor about 2 inches to the right of the hip bone. Walk your right leg straight back behind you allowing the top of the foot to rest on the floor. Square your hips forward and come down onto your forearms. Take 5–8 full breaths, allowing the exhales to be long, slow, and smooth. If you find that you are collapsing onto your left hip, place a blanket underneath your left buttock. (See photo) After completing the pose on the left side, curl your back toes under and press into your hands. Lift your hips up and come into downward facing dog. Bring the right knee forward and do the second side of the pose. After completing the second side of the pose, curl your back toes under and press into your hands. Lift your hips up and come into downward facing dog. Walk your feet up to meet your hands and come up to a standing position at the front of your mat.

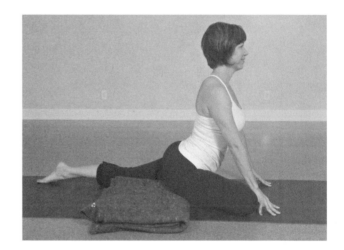

Why Do This?

Pigeon pose is a great hip opener that stretches the outer hip rotators, groins, and thighs as well as the deep abdominal muscles. Opening the hips in this way improves circulation and energy flow through the pelvis.

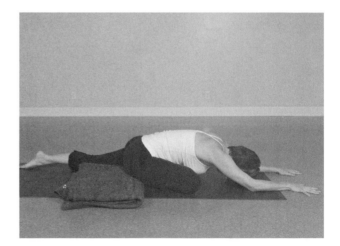

✺ STANDING POSES

10. SIDE ANGLE POSE

Setup

Facing the long side of your mat, step your feet about 3½ to 4 feet apart. Turn your right foot out 90 degrees so that the outer edge of your foot aligns with the side of your mat. Keep your left foot pointing straight ahead or turn it in slightly.

Movement

Bend your right knee towards 90 degrees keeping your knee over your ankle. Check that the kneecap is aligned over the big toe, or even the 2nd toe (NOT to the inside of the big toe). Lean to the right and place your right forearm just above your knee. Place your left hand on your waist and turn your torso toward the sky. Stay here or extend your left arm over your head, keeping the bicep over the ear with the palm facing down. Anchor this forward movement by firmly pressing the outer edge of the back foot into the floor. Take 5–8 breaths. To come up, press down through the feet and legs and bring your torso back up to vertical on an inhale. Pivot the feet so the left foot turns out to 90 degrees and the right foot points straight ahead or turns in slightly. Repeat steps above on the left side.

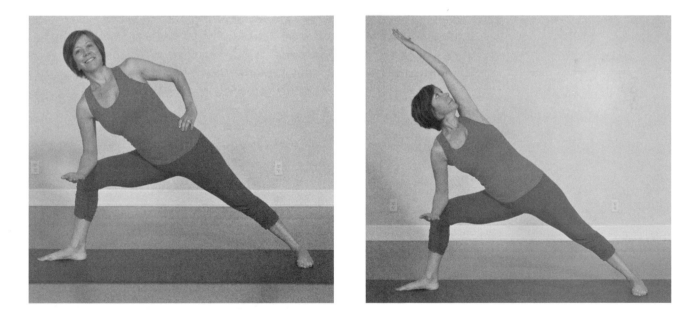

Why Do This?

Side angle pose tones the pelvic organs and can also help with menstrual problems.

11. TRIANGLE POSE

Setup

Facing the long side of your mat, step your feet about 3 ½ to 4 feet apart. Turn your right foot out to the right about 90 degrees, and align the arch of the back foot with the heel of the front foot. Raise your arms parallel to the floor with the palms facing down.

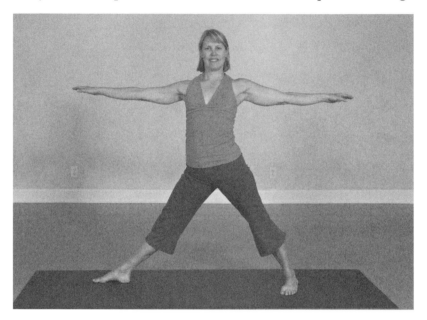

Movement

Exhale and reach out through the right arm, extending your torso forward over the right leg. Bend from the hip joint, not the waist; try to keep the underneath side of the waist long.

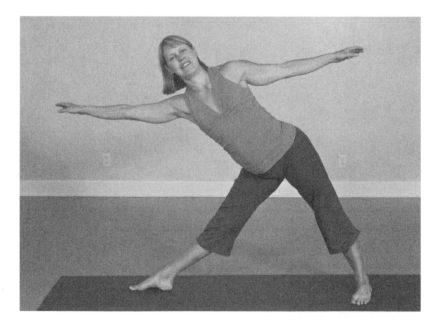

Let your right hand come onto your leg, just letting it rest wherever it comes naturally after reaching out through the right arm. It will likely come to the shin, but possibly to the ankle, or even above the knee joint (don't rest it on the knee joint, though). (Option: use a block underneath the hand, rather than resting the hand on the leg. This adds stability).

Anchor this forward movement by firmly pressing the outer edge of the back foot into the floor. Rotate the ribs toward the ceiling, keeping both the upper and lower sides of the torso equally long. Reach your right arm toward the ceiling, in line with the tops of your shoulders. Keep your head in a position where it feels like the neck is an extension of the rest of the spine. You can look down at the left hand, or look to the right side, or possibly up toward the ceiling. A lower gaze gives more stability. If the neck feels uncomfortable, move it around gently and see if you can find a place where it feels in better alignment. Take 5 to 8 deep breaths. To come up, inhale and imagine that someone is pulling on your top arm to bring you back up to standing. Reverse the feet and repeat for the same length of time on the second side.

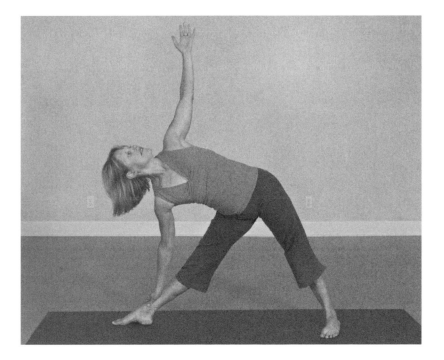

Why Do This?

Triangle pose creates a lot of space in the torso, improving circulation and energy flow through the internal organs and glands.

12. HALF-MOON BALANCE POSE

Setup

Stand in the center of your mat facing the short edge of the mat. Place your feet hip-width (4–6 inches) apart. Step forward with your right foot and take your weight onto your right foot as you allow the right knee to bend a little. Reach your right hand forward, and bring it down to the floor. It should be at least 12 inches in front of the foot, about in line with the little-toe side of the right foot. (Option: use a block underneath the hand; this is easier to reach than the floor).

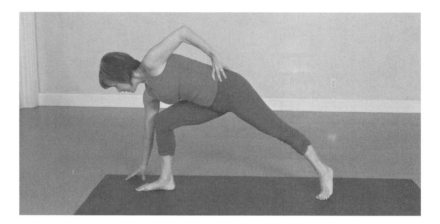

Movement

Begin to straighten your right leg, while lifting the left leg parallel (or a little above parallel) to the floor. Reach back through the left heel to keep the raised leg reaching back strongly. Be careful not to lock or hyperextend the standing knee. Check that the kneecap is aligned over the big toe, or even the 2nd toe (NOT to the inside of the big toe). Most of the weight should be on the foot, not the hand. Rotate your upper torso to the left. *Easiest:* Keep the left hand on the left hip and the eyes gazing down toward the floor near your right hand. *More advanced*: Open the left arm up toward the ceiling, and turn the head to look toward the left. Stay in this position for 3 or more breaths. Then perform the pose standing on the left foot for the same length of time.

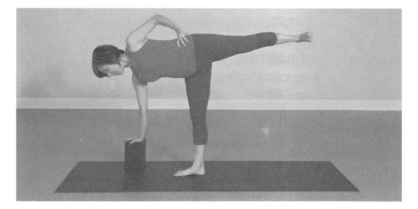

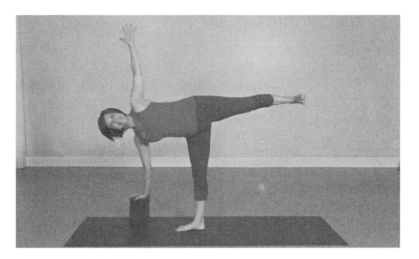

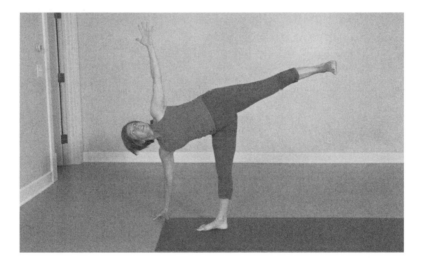

Why Do This?

Half-moon balance pose creates a lot of space in the torso, improving circulation and energy flow through the internal organs and glands.

13. SQUAT POSE AND VARIATIONS

Setup

Stand with feet wider than hip-width apart, approximately 12 inches to start. (The closer your feet are together, the more difficult squat pose is.)

Movement

Bend the knees and lower the sitting bones toward the floor, keeping the back long and the crown of the head up toward the ceiling. The heels should be down on the floor in squat pose. If they don't come to the floor, try taking the feet wider apart or turning the feet out slightly (turning the feet out increases the strain on the knees, though!). If your heels are still off the floor, try one of the variations below. Now, take the palms of the hands together, and press the elbows inside the knees to help open the groin and hips.

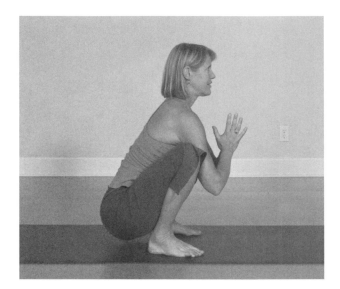

Don't Do This Pose If

If you have knee injuries, squat pose can stress the knee joint. In this case, you can choose the "squat on a block" variation below, or skip squat altogether.

Variations

If you have trouble getting your heels to the floor in squat pose, try one of these options:

1. **Support your heels** on a rolled blanket or yoga mat.

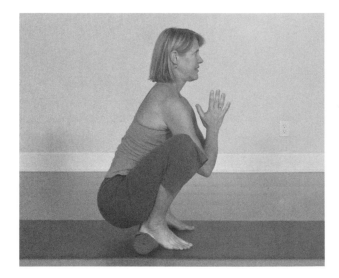

2. **Place your back against a wall.** With feet 12 inches apart, and a few inches away from the wall, slide down the wall to squat pose. If your heels are not on the ground, adjust the distance your feet are from the wall, so that your heels are down. Allow as much of the spine as possible, including the back of the head, to rest back against the wall.

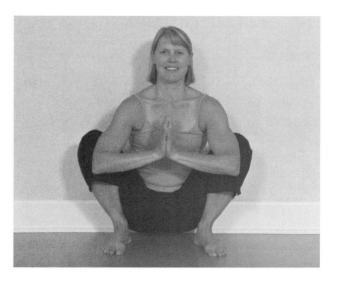

3. **Use a block** underneath the buttocks to support you in squat pose.

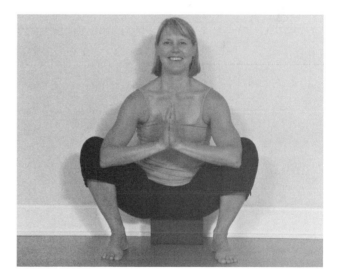

Why Do This?

Squat pose opens the groin, the hips and the pelvic floor, and lengthens the spine. It also strengthens the quadricep muscles along the front of the legs. You may also feel a nice stretch in the low back.

14.   WIDE STANDING FORWARD BEND WITH IMMUNE BOOSTER

Setup

Stand with your feet about 3 feet apart, facing one of the long edges of your mat. Take your hands on your hips. Make sure your feet are parallel to each other.

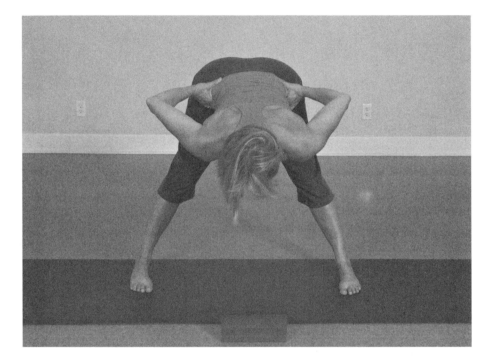

Movement

On an exhale, lean the torso forward from the hip joints. You can bend the knees slightly if your low back feels any strain as you come forward. Release your hands onto the floor directly below your shoulders (or place a block here). Allow the head to release down toward the floor, and take a few breaths here. Then reach the hands behind the back and interweave the fingers together. The backs of the hands should be facing the ceiling, palms toward the back. Keep a slight bend in the elbows, rather than allowing them to hyper-extend. On an inhale, bring the arms up away from the back, and lower toward the back on the exhale. Repeat several times. Then release the hands back down to the floor. Walk the feet towards each other until they are 6 inches or so apart. Bend the knees slightly, let the head and arms hang, and slowly roll up to standing one vertebra at a time. The chin should stay tucked to the chest until you are all the way back to vertical; bring the head up last.

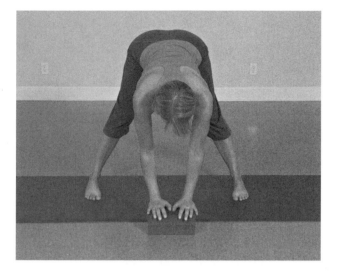

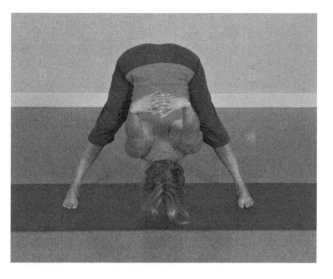

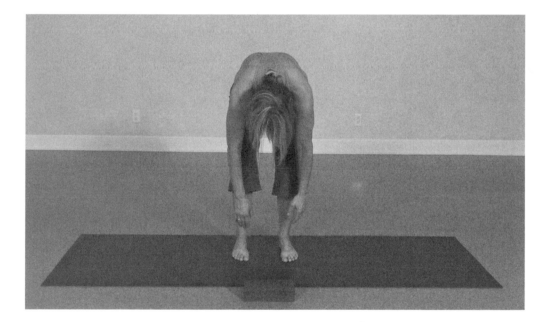

Why Do This?

In addition to the obvious stretch of the hamstrings, forward bends support the endocrine system and help bring hormonal balance to the body. They also tone the organs in the abdominal area, and are calming to the central nervous system. Forward bends raise the yin energy in the body. Taking the arms up and away from the back, with the hands clasped, is an immune system booster, in addition to opening the shoulders.

❀ SEATED POSES

15. FORWARD BEND OVER ONE LEG

Setup

Begin in a seated position with the legs stretched out in front of you. If your lower back feels like it is rounding or your torso is slouching, sit up on a pillow or blanket. This will help to lengthen your spine.

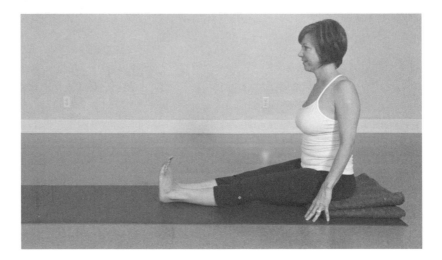

Movement

Bend your left knee and place your left foot into the upper, inner right thigh. Your right leg will stay straight and your right foot will be flexed so that your right toes are facing the sky. Turn your chest and belly over your right thigh and fold forward. Keeping your spine elongated, hold the shin or calf with both hands and take 5 to 8 breaths. If you cannot reach the shin or foot with your hands, use a strap around your right foot. Repeat on the other side.

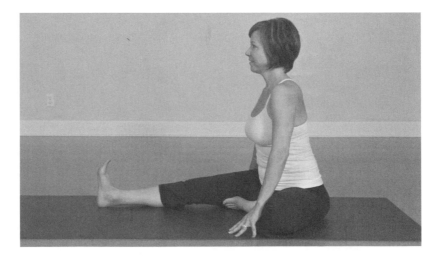

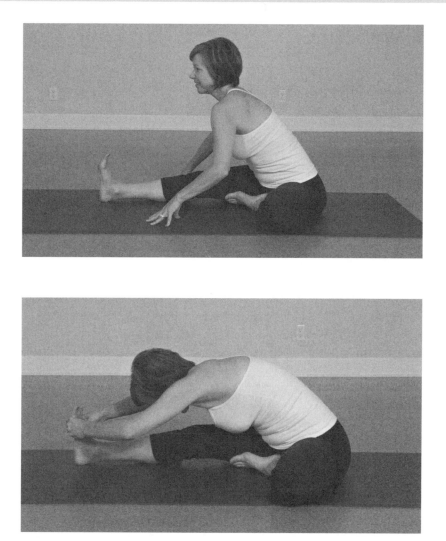

Don't do this pose if there is pain in or around the kneecap of the bent knee. This is a sign of knee stress and an indication that this is not a good position for your knee. Also, don't do this pose if you feel a lot of strain in the low back, which is not relieved by raising the hips on folded blankets.

Why Do This?

This pose calms the nervous system and adrenal glands, and opens the hips. It can help reduce cramps and regulate menstrual flow.

16. COBBLER POSE WITH HEART OPENER

Setup

Begin by sitting on your mat, or raise the hips by sitting on a folded blanket. Take the soles of the feet together, gently allowing the knees to open toward the floor.

Movement

Place your hands behind your hips on the floor in back of you. On an inhale, lengthen your spine and expand your chest while allowing the knees to open gently down toward the floor. On an exhale, roll your shoulders down and back, and open the heart up toward the ceiling. Stay in the pose for 6–8 breaths.

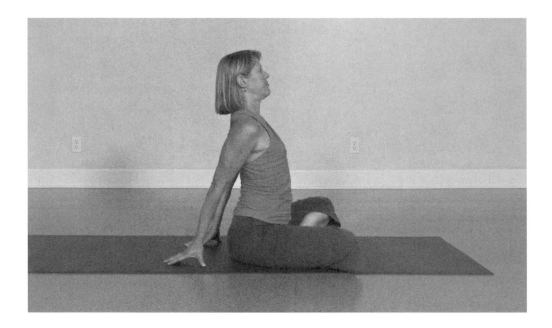

Why Do This?

This pose relaxes the pelvic area, and improves circulation and energy flow in the pelvis and heart center. It releases tension in the upper back and shoulders.

17. SEATED WIDE-LEG STRADDLE

Setup

Sit on a mat or a blanket with the legs apart, feet flexed, toes and knees facing straight up toward the sky. You don't need to take the legs as wide apart as you can, just a comfortable distance apart. Be sure there is a natural curve in the low back. If your back is rounding, place another blanket underneath you.

Movement

Place your hands behind your legs on the floor in back of you. On an inhale, lengthen your spine and expand your chest while pressing the backs of the legs gently down into the floor. You can stay here for 5–8 breaths or you can take the hands in front of you and begin to walk the hands forward, bringing the chest toward the floor. Only go as far forward as your spine allows. You will know you have gone too far if your back begins to round.

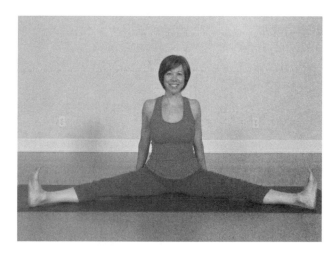
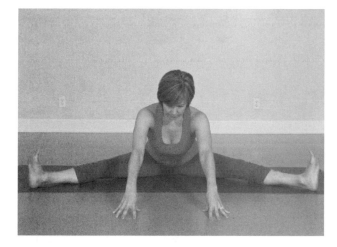

Variation

Turn your chest toward your right leg and fold over the leg. You may want to use a strap around the right foot in this pose. (See photo). Repeat on left side.

Why Do This?

This pose massages the reproductive organs and stimulates the ovaries. It improves circulation in the pelvic floor, and can also help regulate menstrual flow.

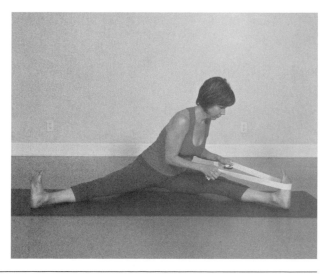

✾ PRE-RELAXATION POSES ON THE BACK

18. PELVIC TILTS

Setup

Lie on your back with the knees bent and feet on the floor hip-width apart (about 4–6 inches apart).

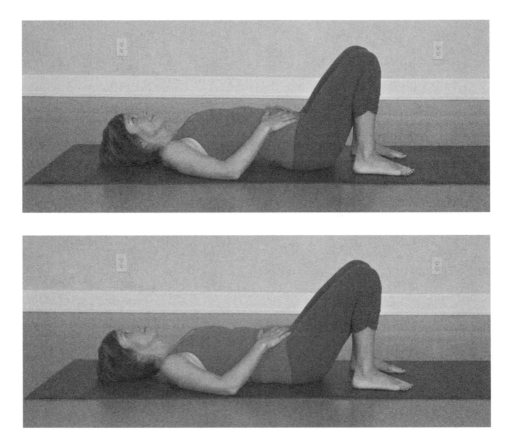

Movement

With an exhale, *gently* press the low back down into the floor. The pubic bone will tilt up toward the navel. On the inhale release and let the low back come up off the floor again. Repeat for 5 to 8 breaths.

Why Do This?

While there are versions of this which are used for core strengthening, that is not our purpose here. We are using this pose to create a gentle rocking of the pelvis. This encourages blood and energy flow, and releases tension and stagnation in the pelvis. For this purpose, press the low back down *gently*, trying not to engage the abdominal muscles any more than necessary to get the action to happen.

19. **BRIDGE POSE

Setup

Setup is the same as for **Pelvic Tilts**. Let your palms rest on the floor on either side of your hips.

Movement

On an inhale, press both feet and hands into the floor and lift the hips straight up toward the sky. Lift and open the heart and try to bring your shoulder blades towards each other. Gently press the back of the head into the floor. Take 5 to 8 breaths. To come out of the pose, on an inhale, take your arms up past your head on the floor. Exhale and lower your body down slowly, from the upper back to the low back and hips. Try to roll down one vertebra at a time. **Don't do this pose during the main flow days of your period.**

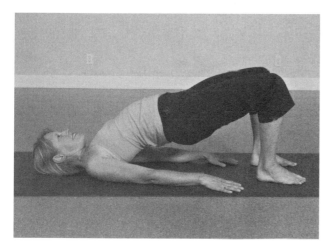
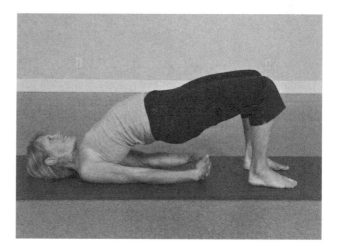

Variation

Instead of pressing your hands into the floor, clasp your hands underneath your back and try to draw the wrists down toward the floor.

Why Do This?

Bridge pose releases tension in the low back and brings energy and vitality to the reproductive organs. It is also opens the heart, releases tension in the neck and shoulders, and helps to regulate the thyroid gland.

20.   BENT KNEE TWIST (SECOND HALF VERSION)

Setup

With your knees bent and feet on the floor, take the feet to the outer edges of your yoga mat. The feet will be about two feet apart. Now, take the arms out to the sides like a "T," with your palms facing up.

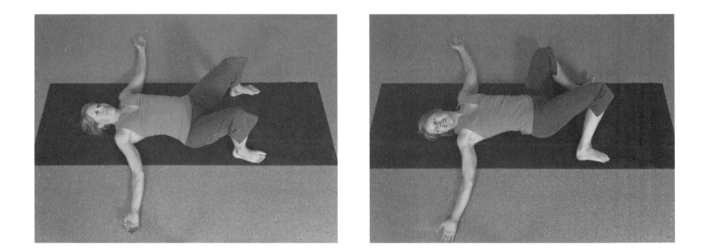

Movement

Lift the hips and shift them slightly toward the left. Then allow the knees to drop over toward the right, keeping the feet touching the mat. You don't need to keep the entire sole of the foot on the floor; it can be the edge of the foot that is still touching the floor. Turn the head to look back toward the left palm. Take 4 or 5 slow, even breaths. On an inhale, bring the knees back to center, and do the twist to the second side.

Why Do This?

Twists are cleansing and rejuvenating for the organs (such as the uterus and intestines) and glands (such as the ovaries and adrenal glands) in the abdominal area. Twists have a calming effect on the central nervous system.

✸ RELAXATION POSES

21. **LEGS UP THE WALL POSE (WITH VARIATIONS)

Set up

Do this pose at a clear space of wall, where you have room to take your legs straight up the wall without bumping into anything. Before you start, put on warm clothes and socks, and have a blanket handy which you can pull over yourself once you get into the pose. Place your yoga mat lengthwise to the wall.

Movement

Start by sitting sideways at the wall, with your right hip just next to the wall and your knees bent. Place your left hand on the floor next to your left hip, and your right hand on the floor behind you. Lean back, and take some weight onto your hands. You might even come down onto your elbows. Next, swing your legs up the wall, so that your sitting bones end up fairly close to the wall. The actual "best" distance from the wall depends partly on your hamstring flexibility. (If your hamstrings are tight, it may help to place a folded blanket on the mat next to the wall, and sit on the blanket to start. Or, take the sitting bones a little further from the wall.) The hands can rest on the low belly, or on either side of you about 12 inches away from the body, with the palms facing up toward the ceiling. This is a resting pose, so make yourself as comfortable as possible. Take care not to get chilled as you are resting. **Don't do this pose during the main flow days of your period.

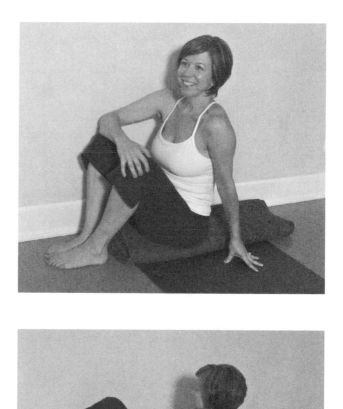

Variations

Try varying the leg position by taking them wider apart, or taking the soles of the feet together like Cobbler Pose. When you get ready to come out of the pose, draw the knees into the chest and roll onto your right side with your knees bent. Rest for a few breaths before using both hands to press up to a seated position.

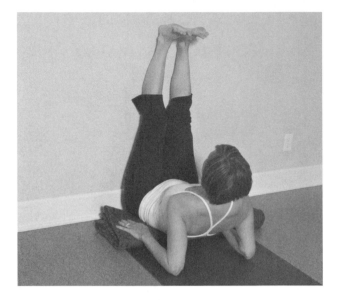

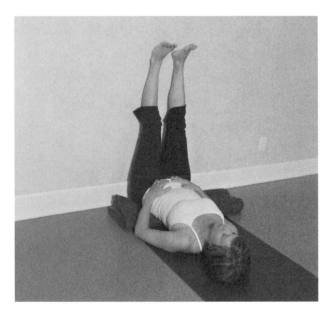

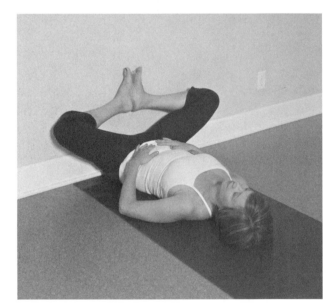

Why Do This?

You may feel like you are doing nothing once you get into the pose, but don't be fooled. This pose is one of the most powerful fertility-supporting yoga poses that you can practice. The abdominal organs are nourished and revitalized when the blood from the feet and legs pools in the low belly. Toxins are removed from the bloodstream, as the blood flows into the lymph glands in the groin. The central nervous system is calmed and the endocrine system is regulated. It is a great pose to do just before bedtime, as it promotes restful sleep. This pose should be done daily for at least 5 minutes, during every part of the cycle except when you are menstruating. You may want to choose one of the visualizations from Chapter 7 to do while you are in this pose.

22. CORPSE POSE

Setup

Lie on your back with your feet and legs relaxed and slightly apart. Allow your arms to rest by your sides a few inches away from your body with your palms facing up. If you have tension or pain in your lower back, place a rolled up blanket or bolster underneath your knees. For added relaxation, place an eye pillow over your eyes.

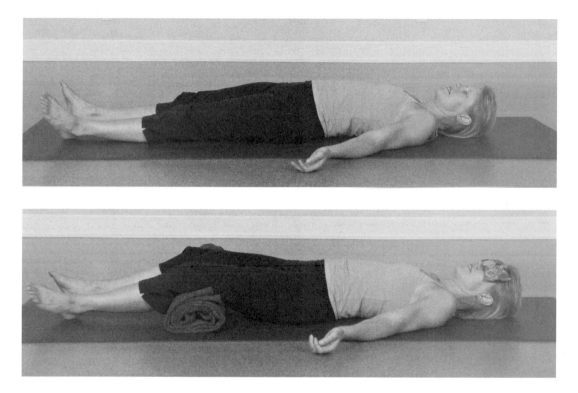

Movement

Feel the support of the floor beneath you, and with each exhale allow your body to feel heavy and relaxed. There is no effort needed here. Tuck your chin ever so slightly toward your chest so the back of the neck is long. Relax and open your palms toward the sky, ready to receive the gifts of your practice. If your mind begins to wander, acknowledge that tendency and let the thoughts come and go with each breath. Stay in this pose for 5–7 minutes or even longer if you have time.

Why Do This?

Corpse pose allows all of the benefits of your practice to integrate into your body, mind and spirit. It can help relieve stress and mild depression, and lower blood pressure. Corpse pose can help with insomnia, fatigue and headaches. It also encourages the mind to rest, as the body sinks into a state of deep relaxation.

6

Yoga Routines for Additional Situations

YOGA DURING YOUR PERIOD

Various opinions exist about how much yoga one should do during the flow days of your period. Some teachers suggest just doing restorative poses during those days. Our take is that you can do as much as is comfortable, although a strenuous practice is not recommended. In addition, there are some categories of poses that are never recommended during your period, including inversions, strong backbends, poses on the belly, abdominal strengthening poses, pelvic floor exercises, and partial inversions such as bridge pose.

The basic idea is that your period is a time to rest and restore. From the yogic perspective, women are fortunate to have periods, which are viewed as an opportunity to cleanse and renew the blood. It is even postulated that this is one reason that women generally live longer than men: these monthly cleansings are important for maintaining health. While you are trying to conceive, the arrival of your period can be a discouraging event. Try reminding yourself that it is an opportunity for your system to cleanse and renew, and make a fresh start. This may help to bring some positive perspective on getting your period.

Below is a short routine that you can safely practice during your period. You can do the whole routine, or you could choose any poses from this routine to do, if you feel like doing less or don't have a lot of time to practice.

✽ YOGA ROUTINE FOR YOUR PERIOD

I. CENTERING/CALMING BREATH (BELLY BREATH)

Setup

This breath can be performed either seated or lying down. Lie down on your back on your mat with your legs straight, or bend the knees if that is more comfortable for the low back. Another option is to sit in a chair with a solid seat that will allow you to sit with a long spine. Let your body relax and place your hands on your low belly.

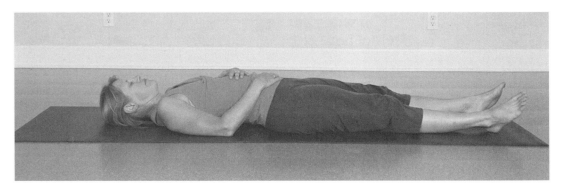

Movement

Breathe fully and deeply into your abdominal region, visualizing the prana (life force energy) filling your belly and creating the loving, open space for life. On the exhalations, visualize stress, defeating thoughts, frustration, etc. all leaving the body. Feel the muscles relax and get heavy with each exhalation. On the inhalations, invite the prana into every cell of your body and feel your hands rise with your breath. Let the gentle rhythm of your breath take you deeper and deeper into relaxation. You may be feeling sad or angry if your period signals that another month has passed without a pregnancy. Allow yourself to notice whatever feelings arise as you are breathing, then simply allow them to release out again with the exhale. Allow yourself to feel gratitude for the cleansing of your system, and the miracle of your cycle. Continue this breathing until you feel calm, and the breath is smooth and even. Ideally, the inhale and exhale should be either equal in length, or the exhale should be a little longer. Allow there to be a bit of a pause at the end of the exhale, and the end of the inhale, before you start the next breath. This "space" is perhaps the most important part of the breath. Try at least 12 full inhales and exhales, but feel free to do more if your mind hasn't calmed after 12 breaths.

Why Do This?

This centering/calming breathing technique helps the body and mind relax. The deep, conscious breaths send signals to the nervous system that the muscles in the body can relax. This is a wonderful way to begin your yoga practice. It can also be used on its own as a technique that can be used any time you need to relax.

❋ POSES LYING ON YOUR BACK

2. SACRUM CIRCLES

Setup

Lie on your back, bend the knees and take the feet up off the floor.

Movement

Put the hands onto the knees and gently circle the knees one direction, keeping an even breath going with the circles. Try to have the movement follow the lead of the breath. After a few circles, pause and switch directions.

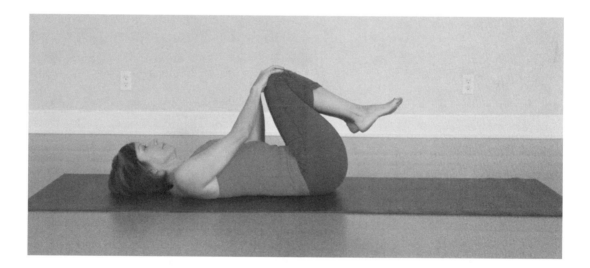

Why Do This?

This action massages the sacrum, which is the flat bone on the low back, at the lower end of the spine. In the yoga "map" of the body, the sacrum is part of the reproductive energy center, so keeping circulation and energy moving through this area is important. This pose helps release low back tension which can accompany your period.

3.   BENT KNEE TWIST (GENTLE VERSION)

Setup

Remain on your back with your knees bent and feet on the floor. Take the feet to the outer edges of your yoga mat. The feet will be about two feet apart. Now, take the arms out to the sides like a "T," with your palms facing up.

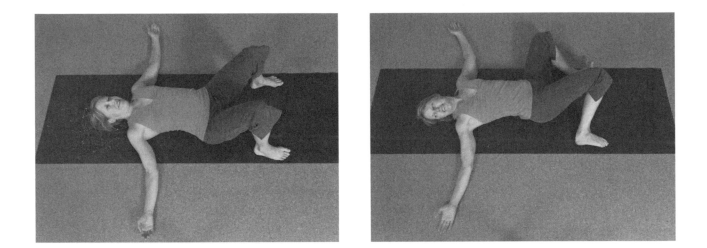

Movement

Lift the hips and shift them slightly toward the left. Then allow the knees to drop slowly over toward the right, keeping the feet touching the mat. You don't need to keep the entire sole of the foot on the floor; it can be the edge of the foot that is still touching the floor. Turn the head to look back toward the left palm. Take 4–5 slow, even breaths. On an inhale, bring the knees back to center, and do the twist to the second side.

Why Do This?

Twists are cleansing and rejuvenating for the organs (such as the uterus and intestines) and glands (such as the ovaries) in the abdominal area. Twists have a calming effect on the central nervous system. During your period, gentle twists aid the cleansing process; however, strenuous twists are not advised.

4. COMING UP

Setup

To prepare for the next set of poses, bend your knees and roll onto your right side. Take a breath or two on your right side.

Movement

Use both hands to gently press yourself back up to a seated position.

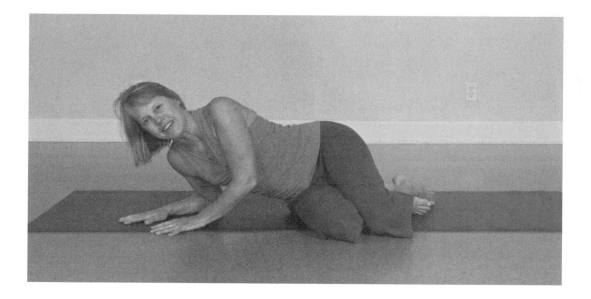

Why Do This?

Rolling to the side and pressing the floor inhibits tension in the neck and lower back. Rolling to the right side keeps the heart on top, so that you don't compress the heart (which is located on the left side). It also keeps the pulse regular, and frees up the breath through the left nostril, which promotes relaxation.

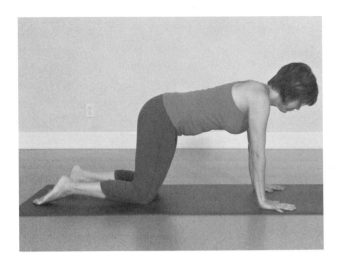

POSES ON HANDS AND KNEES

5. CAT-COW

Setup

Come onto your hands and knees with your wrists underneath your shoulders and your knees underneath your hips. Spread the fingers wide apart from each other. Your knees should be about 4–6 inches apart. If this position bothers your knees, you can try folding a blanket and placing it underneath your knees for extra padding.

Movement

On an inhale, tilt your tailbone up and arch your back. Look forward and draw the shoulders back away from the ears. Keep your core engaged as you arch the back. On an exhale, tilt your tailbone down toward the floor and round your spine. Press the shoulder blades up toward the ceiling. Let your head and neck feel heavy. Repeat at least 5 times, initiating each movement at the tailbone. Allow the movement to follow the breath.

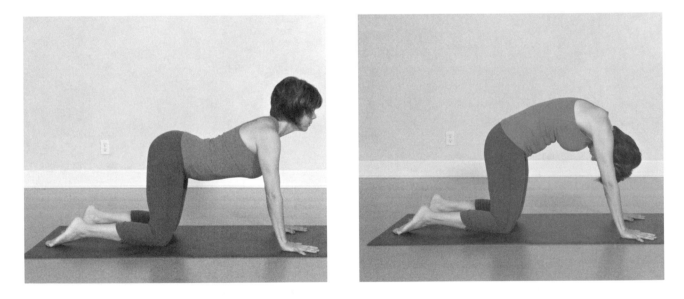

Why Do This?

Cat-cow warms up all of the muscles in the back and allows tension in the neck and shoulders to release. It also opens the major energy channels in the front and back of the body. The pelvic movements can help to relieve menstrual cramps and low back tension.

6. CAT-COW CIRCLES

Setup

Setup is the same as for Cat-Cow.

Movement

Circle the hips and ribcage around to the right, bending the elbows as much as you need to. This is a very free-form movement, so just do what feels good to your body. You may get some forward-and-back movement as well as the circling. Don't forget to breathe while performing these circles. After a few breaths, switch directions.

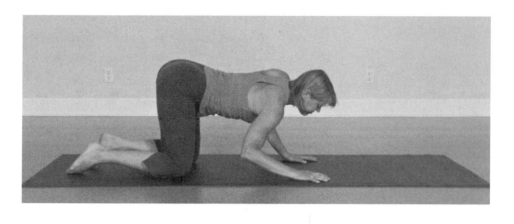

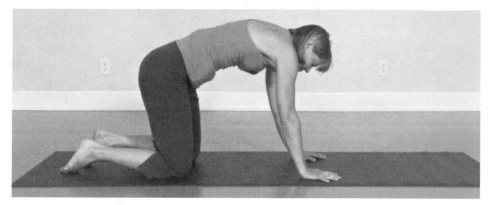

Why Do This?

The circling motion releases tension in the pelvis, ribcage and shoulders. We are taking the torso through a range of motion that most of us don't experience in our regular daily lives, so it encourages us to release physical and emotional patterns where we may be "stuck."

7. PRAYER POSE (CHILD'S POSE)

Setup

From your hands and knees position, take the knees wide apart and sit the hips back onto the heels. Keep the toes together. Bring the forehead to the floor, and reach the arms forward with the palms facing down. If it isn't comfortable to bring the forehead all the way to the floor, you can stack the hands one on top of the other, and rest the forehead on the hands, or rest the forehead on a block or a folded blanket. Let the toes release.

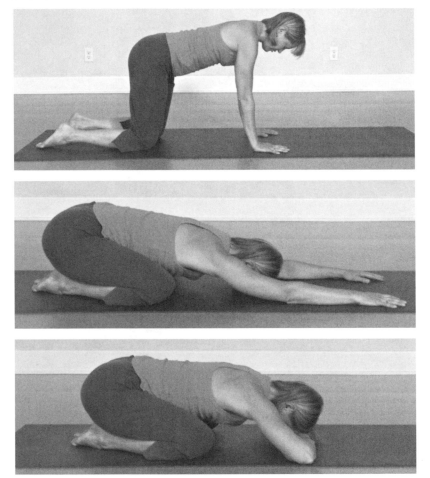

Movement

Prayer pose is a resting pose, so in the standard version of prayer pose, you are resting here, rather than moving. To come up from prayer pose, just walk the hands back in toward the body, and come up slowly.

Why Do This?

Prayer pose is known for its calming effect, which is partly due to resting the forehead down. It also stretches and relaxes the low back and opens the shoulders.

SEATED POSES

8. "CHICKEN WING" SHOULDER STRETCH

Setup

Come to a comfortable seated, cross-legged position. You may want to sit up on the edge of a folded blanket. Take your hands onto your shoulders with the fingers forward, thumbs behind, elbows out to the sides.

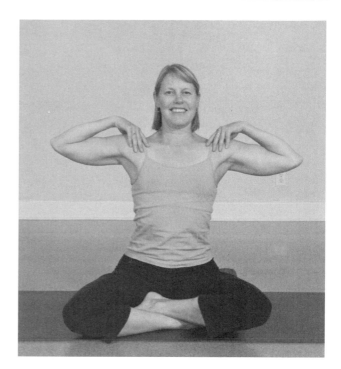

Movement

Inhale and raise the elbows up toward the ceiling. Shrug the shoulders slightly and lengthen the sides of the body. Exhale audibly, through the mouth, lowering the arms back to your sides. Repeat.

Why Do This?

This pose reduces shoulder tension, and opens and lengthens the sides of the body, improving blood flow and energy flow. Audible exhales help clear energy blockages in the throat center, which in turn helps release pelvic tension.

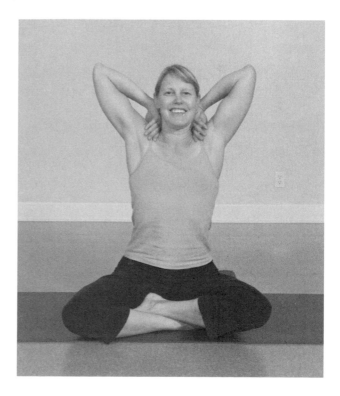

9. SEATED WIDE-LEG STRADDLE

Setup

Sit on a mat or a folded blanket with the legs apart, feet flexed, toes and knees facing straight up. You don't need to take the legs as wide apart as you can, just a comfortable distance apart. Be sure there is a natural curve in the low back. If your back is rounding, add another blanket underneath you.

Movement

Place your hands on the floor behind you. On an inhale, lengthen your spine and expand your chest while pressing the backs of the legs down into the floor. You can stay here for 5–8 breaths or you can take the hands in front of you, and begin to walk the hands forward, bringing the chest toward the floor. Only go as far forward as your spine allows. You will know you have gone too far if your back begins to round.

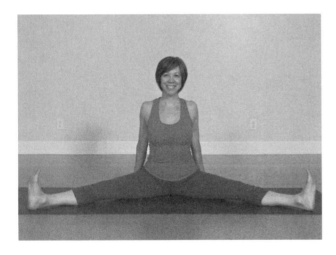
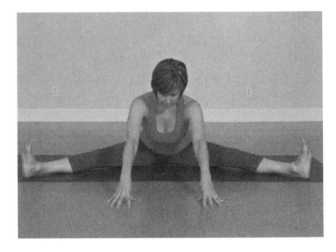

Variation

Turn your chest toward your left leg and stretch toward that leg. You may want to use a strap around the left foot in this pose. Repeat on right side.

Why Do This?

This pose massages the reproductive organs and stimulates the ovaries. It can also help regulate menstrual flow. As with all forward bending poses, this is a calming pose.

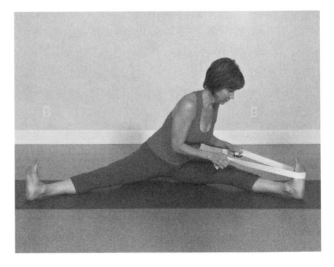

10. COBBLER POSE

Setup

Sitting on your mat, or folded blanket, take the soles of the feet together, gently allowing the knees to open toward the floor.

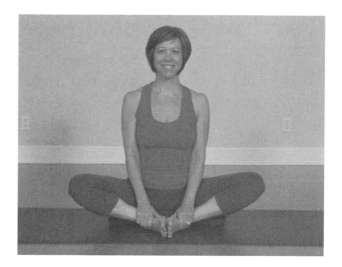

Movement

Place your hands behind your hips on the floor in back of you. On an inhale, lengthen your spine and expand your chest while allowing the knees to open gently down toward the floor. On an exhale, roll your shoulders down and back. You can stay here for 5–8 breaths, or you can take your hands to your feet, bringing the chest down towards the floor. Only go as far forward as your spine allows. You will know you have gone too far if your back begins to round.

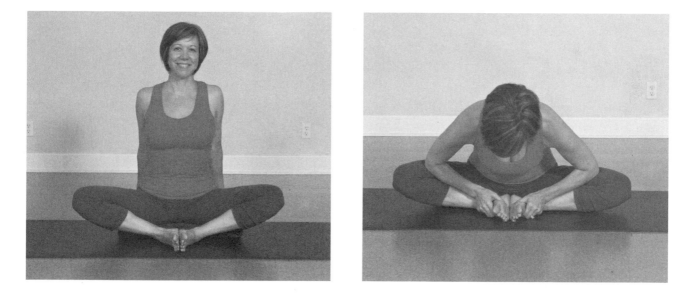

Why Do This?

This pose relaxes the pelvic area, and improves energy flow and blood circulation in the pelvis. This is one of the best poses to counter menstrual cramps.

11. GENTLE SEATED TWIST

Setup

Sit on your mat or folded blanket in a comfortable, cross-legged position, as for the Chicken Wing Pose. As you do the twist, be aware of keeping the spine straight and long.

Movement

On an inhale, reach down through the sitting bones, and up through the crown of the head. Take your right hand onto your left knee, and place your left hand behind you on the floor or on the blanket. The hand placement should be just a few inches behind you—not so far behind that you need to lean back to put the hand down. On the exhale, begin to twist to the left. This should be a gentle twist, so only take the turn to about 90 degrees. Try turning first with the belly, then the shoulder, and finally following with the head, keeping the movement smooth. Keep the chin level as you turn. On your next inhale, back out of the twist slightly, lengthen the spine, and with the exhale twist again. Try to keep both sitting bones down as you turn. Reverse the hands and twist to the second side.

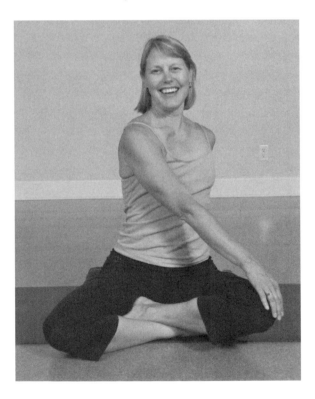 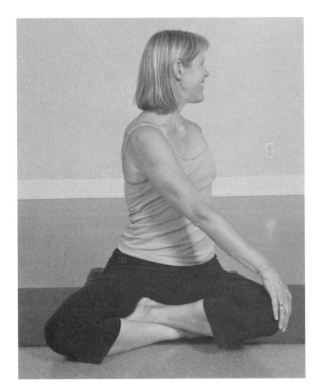

Why Do This?

This twist massages the abdominal organs, including the uterus and ovaries. It also balances energy in the body, reduces stress, and relieves tension in the low back, neck and mid-back.

✿ RELAXATION POSES

12. RECLINED COBBLER POSE

Setup

Sit on the mat with your legs comfortably crossed and a bolster right behind you. Have the bolster close enough so that your sacrum is touching it. If you don't have a bolster, you can make one by rolling your yoga mat in a folded blanket, and propping one end of this roll up on your block.

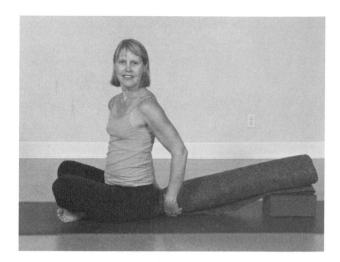

Movement

Bend your knees and bring the soles of the feet onto the mat and your hands on the mat next to your hips. Begin to slowly lower yourself back onto the bolster or blanket roll until your entire back and head are supported. (If you are not using any props, then simply lie back on the floor with the knees bent, soles of the feet on the floor). Bring the soles of the feet together to touch, and slowly allow your knees to release toward the floor. You can place cushions or folded blankets under your thighs for additional support. Rest your hands on your belly, or allow them to gently rest by your sides, palms facing up. Stay in this pose for up to 10 minutes if time allows. Come out if the hips or knees feel any discomfort.

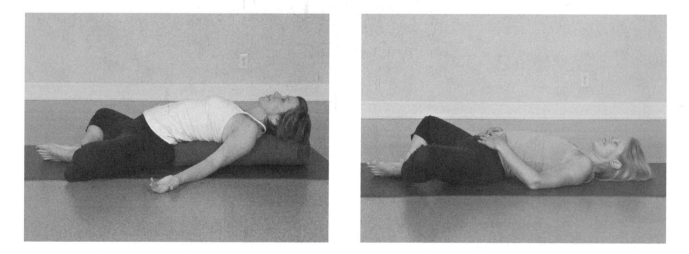

Why Do This?

This pose helps the abdomen and lower back to relax. It allows for a gentle opening of the hips and can help alleviate menstrual pain. Sometimes referred to as "goddess pose," this pose is wonderful for helping the apana energy flow downwards, especially during menstruation.

YOGA FOR EARLY PREGNANCY

If you get a positive pregnancy test, congratulations! This is also an important time to keep up a gentle yoga practice, to support the early pregnancy. Yoga helps maintain a healthy uterus, and also helps to keep you calm. Recent studies have shown that the effects on the baby of stress while in utero can be life-long. Taking good care of yourself and keeping stress levels low during pregnancy is critical, and yoga is one of the best ways to accomplish this.

During early pregnancy, any of the poses in our Second Half Basic Routine are appropriate and are useful to do. Please note that **Legs up the Wall** is still a very important pose to support the pregnancy, but we generally recommend the following modification during first trimester:

LEGS UP THE COUCH POSE (LEGS UP THE WALL WITH MODIFICATIONS FOR EARLY PREGNANCY)

Setup

Before you start, put on warm clothes and socks, and have a blanket handy which you can pull over yourself once you get into the pose. Place your yoga mat lengthwise to your couch, or to a chair.

Movement

Start by sitting sideways with your right hip just next to the front of the chair or couch, and your knees bent. Place your left hand on the floor next to your left hip, and your right hand on the floor behind you. Lean back, taking some weight onto your hands. You might even come down onto your right elbow. Next, swing your legs up onto the seat of the chair or couch, so that your legs are bent at about a 90 degree angle. The hands can rest on the low belly, which creates a connection from your heart center to the baby. You may want to use this time to send positive messages to the baby. Or, take this time to tune into your body's own

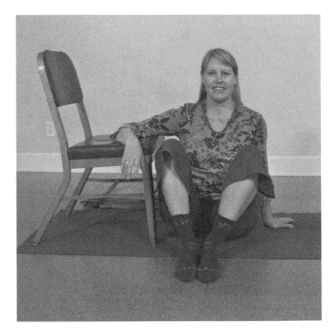

wisdom that has allowed this pregnancy to happen, and is guiding the process of pregnancy and birth. This is a resting pose, so make yourself as comfortable as possible. Take care not to get chilled as you are resting. Stay in the pose at least 5 minutes. When you get ready to come out of the pose, draw the knees into the chest and roll onto your right side with your knees bent. Rest for a few breaths on your side, before using both hands to press up to a seated position.

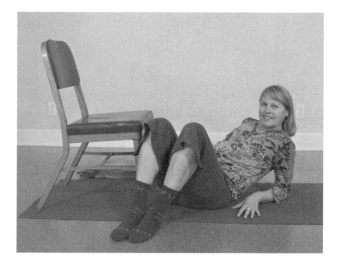

Why Do This?

The uterus is nourished when the blood from the feet and legs pools in the low belly. This helps to create a supportive environment in the uterus for the fetus to grow. In addition, the central nervous system is calmed and the endocrine system is regulated. During later pregnancy, this pose helps to alleviate swelling in the feet, ankles and legs. It is a great pose to do just before bedtime, as it promotes restful sleep. This pose should be done daily for at least 5 minutes, unless lying down exacerbates nausea or heartburn.

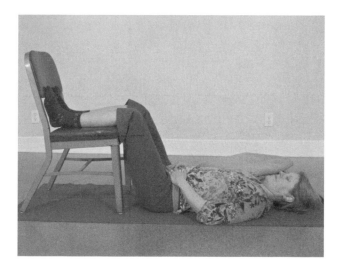

✳ CYCLES USING ASSISTED REPRODUCTIVE TECHNOLOGY (ART)

The following yoga practice is designed for anyone who is going through fertility treatments or is feeling stressed out from the challenge of trying to conceive. While the poses are great for fertility, they are also geared especially toward calming and relaxing the central nervous system. You can do the entire routine if time allows, or just choose one or two restorative poses. You can stay in each pose for up to ten minutes. You may want to play soft music or a guided meditation, or simply enjoy the peace and quiet while you practice.

If you are working with a fertility clinic using assisted reproductive technology (ART), you can continue doing yoga during your ART cycle, as long as your doctor approves. You will need to modify the poses based on what phase of ART you are in. We strongly recommended that you have the supervision of a fertility yoga instructor during ART. If this is not possible, you may follow the basic guidelines set out in the box below. Please note that during the "stim" phase of the ART cycle (while doing injectable drugs for ovary stimulation), it is important to immediately stop any pose that feels uncomfortable. Avoid twisting or doing any poses that create pressure on the low belly. You may also need to modify your yoga poses based on how the stim phase is progressing. For example, if your doctor says you need to reduce the dosage of the stim drugs you are taking, or says you are stimming "too fast," then you should stop doing **Legs up the Wall Pose**. If your doctor increases your dosage of stim drugs, or says things are not progressing as well as they had hoped, then you should increase the time you spend in **Legs up the Wall Pose**. In this case, try doing the pose twice a day for 5–10 minutes each time.

POSE SCHEDULE FOR IVF CYCLE

Until period starts

All poses from Second Half Routines

During period

No abdominal strengthening poses
No poses on belly
No pelvic floor contractions
No Legs Up the Wall Pose
No inversions or partial inversions
Do the *Yoga Routine for Your Period* at the beginning of this chapter (if comfortable)

During suppression (on birth control or lupron)

All poses from either First or Second Half Routines

During stimulation phase (using injectables); please also read preceding paragraph:

No poses on belly after Day 5 of Stim drugs (or sooner if it gets uncomfortable and/or you feel bloated)

Limit twisting: *gentle* twists only

No abdominal strengthening poses; no inversions

No strenuous poses of any kind

Stop any pose that gets uncomfortable

Between retrieval and transfer

Any Second Half poses after initial rest day, as long as poses are comfortable

Post transfer

Initially, take 3 rest days doing only **belly breathing, Legs Up the Wall Pose, Reclined Cobbler Pose or Supported Bridge Pose**.

After 3 days, you can add back any other Second Half Poses that feel comfortable, as long as your doctor approves.

YOGA ROUTINE FOR ART CYCLES OR STRESS RELIEF

I. CALMING/CENTERING BREATH (BELLY BREATH)

Setup

This breath can be performed either seated or lying down. Lie on your back on your mat with your legs straight, or bend the knees if that is more comfortable for the low back. Another option is to sit in a chair with a solid seat that will allow you to sit with a long spine. Let your body relax and place your hands on your low belly.

Breathe fully and deeply into your abdomen. Imagine prana (life force energy) filling your belly on each inhale, and creating the loving, open space for life. On the exhalations, visualize stress, defeating thoughts, frustration, etc. all leaving the body. Feel the muscles relax and get heavy with each exhalation. On the inhalations, invite the prana into every cell of your body. Feel your hands rise and fall with your breath. Let the gentle rhythm of your breath take you deeper and deeper into relaxation. Set an intention related to releasing stress, or to being kind to yourself during this process. Continue this breathing until you feel calm, and the breath is smooth and even. Ideally, the inhale and exhale should be either equal in length, or the exhale should be a little longer. Allow there to be a bit of a pause at the end of the exhale, and the end of the inhale, before you start the next breath. This "space" is perhaps the most important part of the breath. Try at least 12 full inhales and exhales, but feel free to do more if your mind hasn't calmed after 12 breaths.

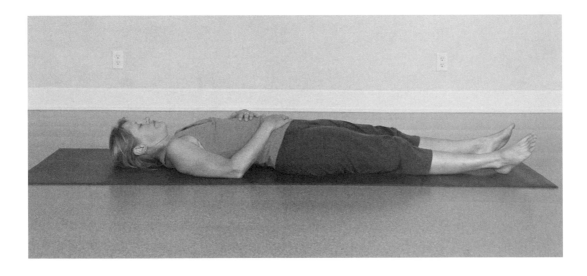

Why Do This?

This centering/calming breathing technique helps the body and mind relax. The deep, conscious breaths send signals to the nervous system that the muscles in the body can relax. This is a wonderful way to begin the practice or a technique that can be used any time you need to relax.

POSES LYING ON YOUR BACK

2. RECLINED COBBLER POSE

Setup

Sit on the mat with your legs comfortably crossed and a bolster right behind you. Have the bolster close enough so that your sacrum is touching it. If you don't have a bolster, you can make one by rolling your yoga mat in a folded blanket, and propping one end of this roll up on your block (see photo).

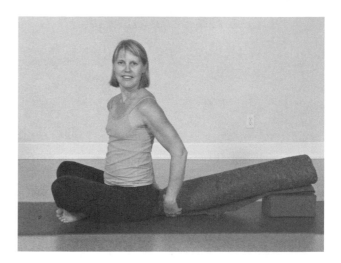

Movement

Bend your knees and bring the soles of the feet onto the mat and your hands on the mat next to your hips. Begin to slowly lower yourself back onto the bolster or blanket roll until your entire back and head are supported. (If you are not using any props, then simply lie back on the floor with the knees bent, soles of the feet on the floor). Bring the soles of the feet together to touch, and slowly allow your knees to release toward the floor. You can place cushions or folded blankets under your thighs for additional support. Rest your hands on your belly, or allow them to gently rest by your sides, palms facing up. Stay in this pose for up to 10 minutes if time allows. Come out if the hips or knees feel any discomfort.

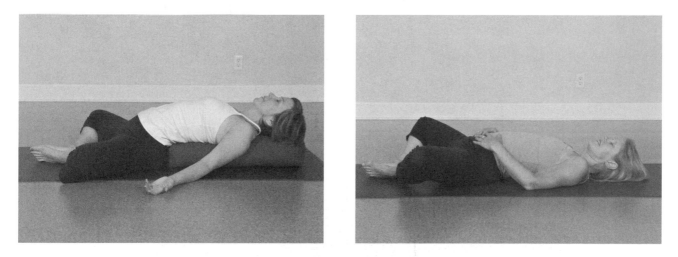

Why Do This?

This pose helps the abdomen and lower back to relax. It allows for a gentle opening of the hips and can help alleviate menstrual pain. Sometimes referred to as "goddess pose," this pose is wonderful for helping the apana flow downwards, especially during menstruation.

✿ POSES ON HANDS AND KNEES

3. CAT-COW

Setup

Come onto your hands and knees with your wrists underneath your shoulders and your knees underneath your hips. Spread the fingers wide apart from each other. Your knees should be about 4–6 inches apart. If this position bothers your knees, you can try folding a blanket and placing it underneath your knees for extra padding.

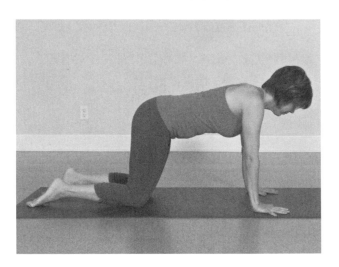

Movement

On an inhale, tilt your tailbone up and arch your back. Look forward and draw the shoulders back away from the ears. Keep your core engaged as you arch the back. On an exhale, tilt your tailbone down toward the floor and round your spine. Press the shoulder blades up toward the ceiling. Let your head and neck feel heavy. Repeat at least 5 times, initiating each movement at the tailbone. Allow the movement to follow the breath.

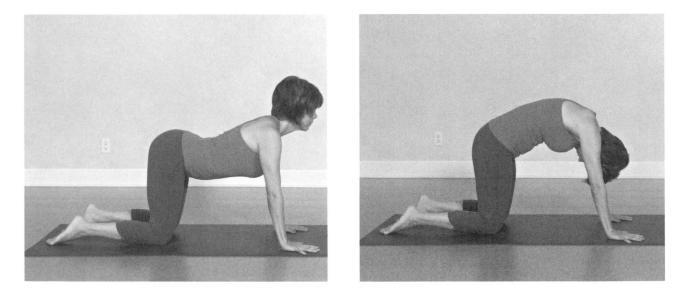

Why Do This?

Cat-cow warms up all of the muscles in the back and allows tension in the neck and shoulders to release. It also opens the major energy channels in the front and back of the body. The pelvic movements bring blood flow and energy through the pelvis.

4. CAT-COW CIRCLES

Setup

Setup is the same as for Cat-Cow.

Movement

Circle the hips and ribcage around to the right, bending the elbows as much as you need to. This is a very free-form movement, so just do what feels good to your body. You may get some forward-and-back movement as well as the circling. Don't forget to breathe while performing these circles. After a few breaths, switch directions.

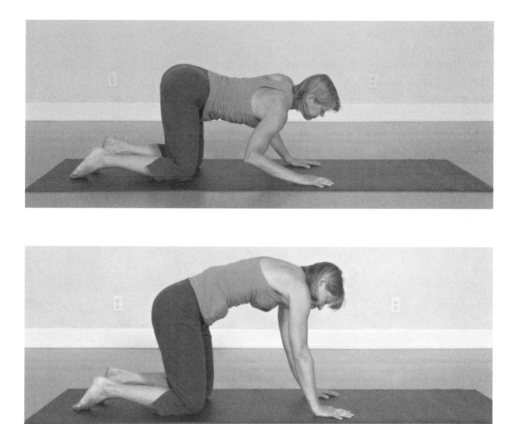

Why Do This?

The circling motion releases tension in the pelvis, ribcage and shoulders. We are taking the torso through a range of motion that most of us don't experience in our regular daily lives, so it encourages us to release physical and emotional patterns where we may be "stuck."

5. RESTORATIVE CHILD'S POSE WITH BOLSTER OR BLANKET STACK

Setup

Come to a kneeling position. Take the knees a bit wider apart, then place a bolster between the knees. (If you don't have a bolster, you can fold a blanket or two into a stack that is about 2 feet wide and about 8–12 inches tall).

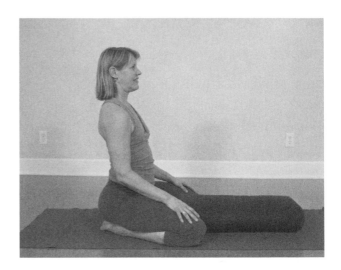

Movement

As you sit the hips back onto the heels, lay your chest and belly onto the bolster or blanket stack. Turn your head to the side, and reach your arms forward with the palms resting down, or gently hold onto the bolster with your hands.

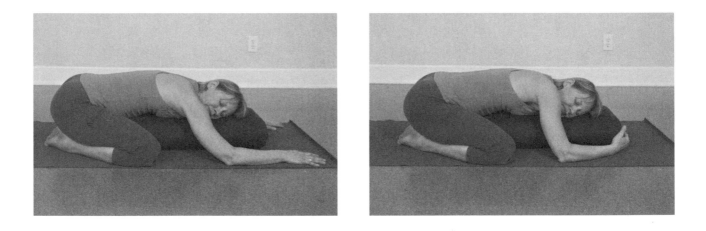

Why Do This?

This is a resting, nurturing pose that supports the front of the body, and allows the hips and legs to gently open while stretching and relaxing the low back. It is also known for its calming effect.

✿ SEATED POSES

6. "CHICKEN WING" SHOULDER STRETCH

Setup

Sit in a comfortable seated, cross-legged position. You may want to sit up on one or two folded blankets if your hips, knees or low back are uncomfortable when sitting on the mat without support. Make sure you are sitting straight down on your sitting bones, not leaning forward or rounding the low back. Take your hands onto your shoulders with the fingers forward, thumbs behind, elbows out to the sides.

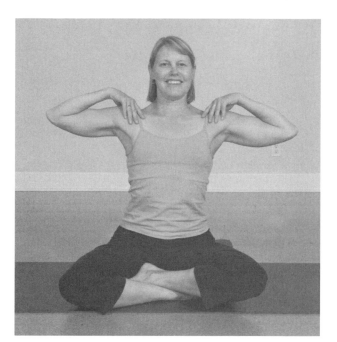

Movement

Inhale and raise the elbows up toward the ceiling. Shrug the shoulders slightly and lengthen the sides of the body. Exhale audibly, through the mouth, lowering the arms back to your sides. Repeat 4–6 times.

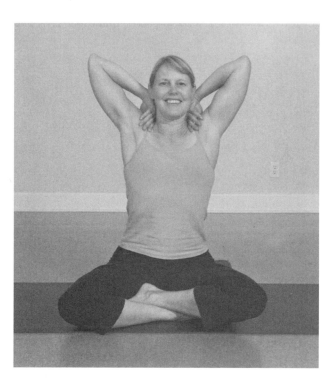

Why Do This?

This pose reduces shoulder tension, and opens and lengthens the sides of the body, improving blood and energy flow. Audible exhales help clear energy blockages in the throat center, which in turn helps release pelvic tension.

7. COBBLER POSE WITH HEART OPENER

Setup

Begin by sitting on your mat, or raise the hips by sitting on a folded blanket. Take the soles of the feet together, gently allowing the knees to open toward the floor.

Movement

Place your hands behind your hips on the floor in back of you. On an inhale, lengthen your spine and expand your chest while allowing the knees to open gently down toward the floor. On an exhale, roll your shoulders down and back, and open the heart up toward the ceiling. Stay in the pose for 6–8 breaths.

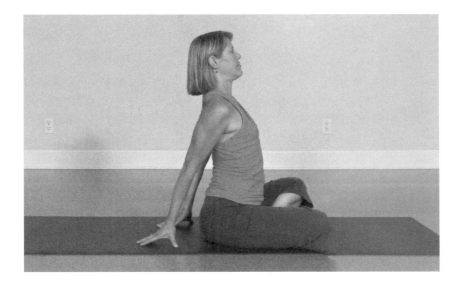

Why Do This?

This pose relaxes the pelvic area, and improves energy flow and blood circulation in the pelvis and heart center. It releases tension in the upper back and shoulders.

✸ MORE POSES LYING ON YOUR BACK

8. **SUPPORTED BRIDGE POSE

Setup

Set your block near your mat. Lie on your back with your knees bent and your feet on the floor, hip-width (4–6 inches apart). Let your palms rest on the floor on either side of your hips.

Movement

On an inhale, press both feet and hands into the floor and lift the hips straight up. Place your block onto the floor just underneath your sacrum, which is the small triangular-shaped bone at the base of the spine. You may have to move the block up or down to find the place that feels most comfortable. Start with the block at the lowest height (widest side on the floor). If you need additional height, you can turn the block to rest on its narrow edge. Your arms can rest by your sides with the palms facing up, or you can place your hands on your belly. Allow your whole body to relax here. You may feel a release in the pelvis and low back. You can stay in this pose for up to 5 minutes. Take at least 10 breaths in the pose with the eyes closed. *Note: If you experience any discomfort in the low back, remove the block and rest on the back.* **Don't do this pose if you are on the main flow days of your period**.

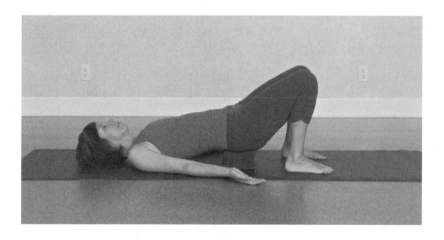

Why Do This?

Supported bridge releases tension in the pelvis and low back, and brings energy and vitality to the reproductive organs. It is also helps to release tension in the neck and shoulders. Because of the slight downward angle, this pose helps to regulate the entire endocrine system. It is also very calming to the central nervous system.

9. KNEES TO CHEST

Setup

Bend your knees and take your feet up off the floor. Place your hands on your knees.

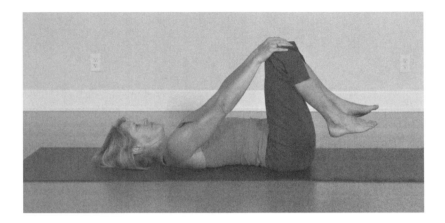

Movement

On an exhale, bring your knees gently toward your chest; don't hug them in, just gently draw them in. On your inhale, push the knees gently away as far as your arms can comfortably reach. The feet will remain off of the floor. Repeat the movement 5 to 8 more times. The focus should be mostly on the breath, rather than on the movement. Move slowly, using the whole exhale to bring the knees toward your chest, and the whole inhale to straighten your arms again.

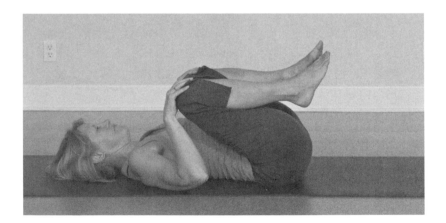

Why Do This?

This movement releases tension in the low back. It also gently compresses the abdominal area, increasing blood flow through that area.

10. OUTER HIP STRETCH (#4 POSE)

Setup

Find your strap. With your knees bent and feet on the floor, lift the left foot, and pass the strap around the left shin. Release the right foot back to the floor. Hold one end of the strap in each hand. Now, cross the right ankle inside the left knee. One end of the strap should come through the triangular space in the center between the two legs.

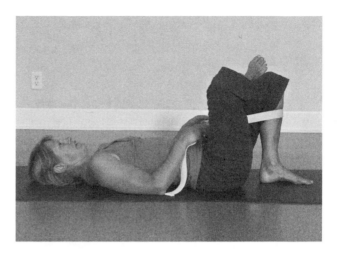

Movement

If you are already feeling a lot of stretch in the right outer hip or hamstring area, just keep the left foot on the floor and breathe. For more stretch, pull on the straps to draw the left knee gently toward the chest. Breathe with full, even breaths. Try 5–8 breaths here. Switch the legs and do the other side of the pose. Let the shoulders relax as much as possible while holding the strap. Relax the face muscles, too. See how many muscles in the body you can relax while allowing the outer hip rotators to stretch. (**modification:** if you have knee injuries, don't take the strap around the shin. Instead, pass the strap under the knee).

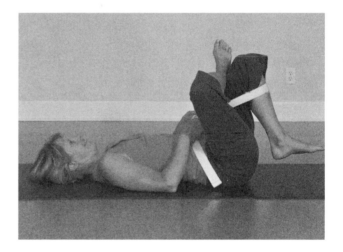

Why Do This?

This pose releases the rotator muscles in the outer hips, which are a group of short, but powerful muscles that are tight on many people. Releasing tension in these muscles also releases tension in the pelvic area, and allows energy and blood flow to move more easily through this area. This stretch also helps alleviate low back problems.

11. BENT KNEE TWIST (GENTLE VERSION)

Setup

Remain on your back, with your knees bent and feet on the floor. Take the feet to the outer edges of your yoga mat. The feet will be about two feet apart. Now, take the arms out to the sides like a "T," with your palms facing up.

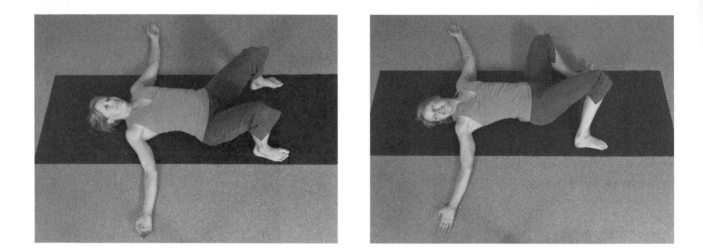

Movement

Lift the hips and shift them slightly toward the left. Then allow the knees to drop slowly over toward the right, keeping the feet touching the mat. You don't need to keep the entire sole of the foot on the floor; it can be the edge of the foot that is still touching the floor. Turn the head to look back toward the left palm. Take several slow, even breaths. On an inhale, bring the knees back to center, and do the twist to the second side.

Why Do This?

Twists are cleansing and rejuvenating for the organs (such as the uterus and intestines) and glands (such as the ovaries) in the abdominal area. Twists have a calming effect on the central nervous system. During an ART cycle, gentle twists such as this one can support the process; however, strenuous twists are not advised. *Note: If you are taking stim drugs and feel any discomfort, refrain from doing even this twist.*

✸ RELAXATION POSES

12.   **LEGS UP THE WALL POSE (WITH VARIATIONS)

Setup

Do this pose at a clear space of wall, where you have room to take your legs straight up the wall without bumping into anything. Before you start, put on warm clothes and socks, and have a blanket handy which you can pull over yourself once you get into the pose. Place your yoga mat lengthwise to the wall.

Movement

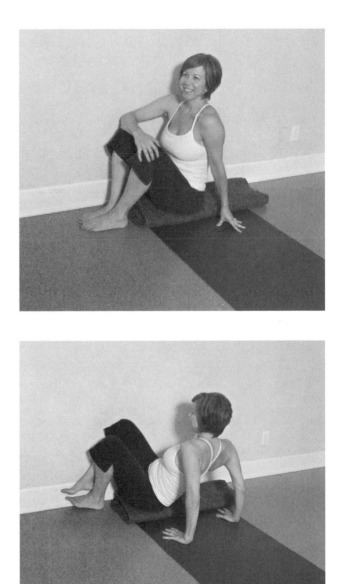

Start by sitting sideways at the wall, with your right hip just next to the wall and your knees bent. Place your left hand on the floor next to your left hip, and your right hand on the floor behind you. Lean back, and take some weight onto your hands. You might even come down onto your elbows. Next, you will need to swing your legs up the wall, so that your sitting bones end up fairly close to the wall. The actual "best" distance from the wall depends partly on your hamstring flexibility. Find a place where your hamstrings are not unhappy when your legs are up the wall. (If your hamstrings are tight, it may help to place a folded blanket on the mat next to the wall, and sit on the blanket to start. Or, take the sitting bones a little further from the wall.) **Don't do this pose during the main flow days of your period**.

Variations

You can keep the legs a few inches apart on the wall, or try varying the leg position by taking them wider apart, or taking the soles of the feet together like Cobbler Pose. The hands can rest on the low belly, or on either side of you about 12 inches away from the body, with the palms facing up toward the ceiling.

This is a resting pose, so make yourself as comfortable as possible. Take care not to get chilled as you are resting. This pose may take a few practice tries, and may feel awkward at first. This is a very important fertility pose—so don't give up. When you get ready to come out of the pose, draw the knees into the chest and roll onto your right side with your knees bent. Rest for a few breaths before using both hands to press up to a seated position.

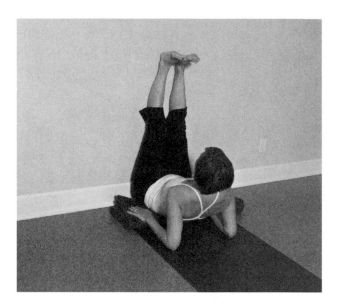

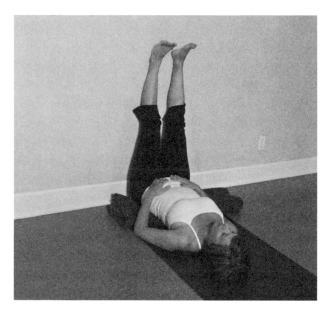

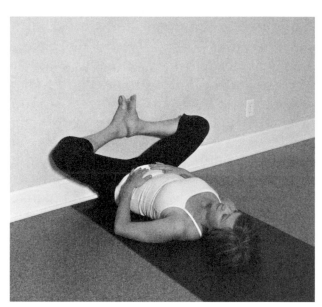

Why Do This?

You may feel like you are doing nothing once you get into the pose, but don't be fooled. This pose is one of the most powerful fertility-supporting yoga poses that you can practice. The abdominal organs are nourished and revitalized when the blood from the feet and legs pools in the low belly. Toxins are removed from the bloodstream, as the blood flows into the lymph glands in the groin. The central nervous system is calmed and the endocrine system is regulated. It is a great pose to do just before bedtime, as it promotes restful sleep. This pose is very important to do during an ART cycle, as it supports the ovary stimulation and builds uterine lining. You may want to choose one of the visualizations from Chapter 7 to do while you are in this pose.

13. CORPSE POSE

Setup

Lie on your back with your feet and legs relaxed and apart. Allow your arms to rest by your sides a few inches away from your body with your palms facing up. If you have tension or pain in your lower back, place a rolled up blanket or bolster underneath your knees. For added relaxation, place an eye pillow over your eyes.

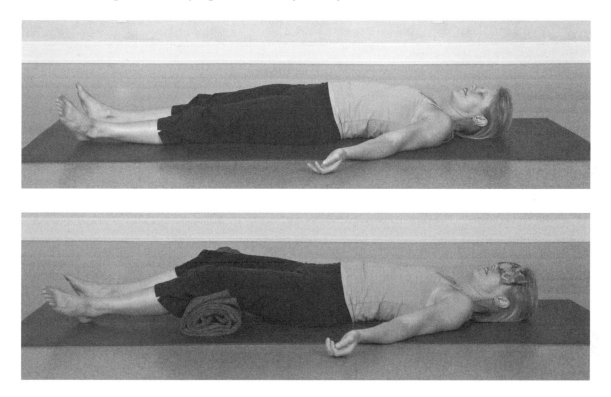

Movement

Feel the support of the floor beneath you, and with each exhale allow your body to feel heavy and relaxed. There is no effort needed here. Tuck your chin ever so slightly toward your chest so the back of the neck is long. Relax and open your palms toward the sky, ready to receive the gifts of your practice. If your mind begins to wander, acknowledge that tendency and let the thoughts come and go with each breath. Stay in this pose for 5–7 minutes or even longer if you have time.

Why Do This?

Corpse pose allows all of the benefits of your practice to integrate into your body, mind and spirit. It can help relieve stress and mild depression, and lower blood pressure. Corpse pose can also help people who suffer from insomnia, fatigue and headaches. It also encourages the mind to rest, as the body sinks into a state of deep relaxation.

✦ ADAPTING YOUR YOGA PRACTICE IN A CLASS

Not every city has a Yoga for Fertility class, and you may enjoy the community and instruction you receive in a class structure. If you are attending a yoga class in a studio or health club while trying to conceive, it is important to choose a class that is gentle, with a practice that is not too strenuous. See Chapter 1 for some suggested types of classes that are more supportive for someone trying to conceive. You may want to read the section of Chapter 8 that talks about exercise and fertility, for additional explanation regarding our recommendations for yoga practice.

If you plan to attend a yoga class while trying to conceive, here are our key recommendations:

MODIFYING YOGA CLASSES WHEN TRYING TO CONCEIVE

- Choose a gentle type of yoga class (not power yoga, or strenuous practices that emphasize moving quickly from one pose to another. Also, avoid practices conducted in over- heated rooms).
- Inform the teacher that you will likely be modifying some poses, and explain why.
- Minimize core work, or abdominal strengthening, in all phases of your cycle.
- Avoid strong breathing (pranayama) practices including kapalabhati or bhastrika, "breath of fire," and breath retention.
- In the first half of your cycle, after your main flow days are finished, you should be okay doing most poses in a gentle class, noting the modifications on core work and breathing practices mentioned above.
- In the second half of your cycle, also avoid strenuous twists, and any poses which increase pressure on your belly, such as Bow Pose.
- During your period, follow the recommendations set out earlier in this chapter regarding modifying your practice during your period: no pelvic floor exercises, no inversions or partial inversions, no poses that compress the belly, no strong backbends; only gentle twists.

Some people find that they are not comfortable attending a class if they are not able to do the poses the way the class is doing them. Or, they find that they push themselves harder than they should in a class setting. If you find that it is too difficult to attend a class and modify poses, then it would be better to just practice on your own, at home, using the routines we have set out in this book, or our Yoga and Fertility DVD.

🌸 YOGA WITH YOUR PARTNER

Although we have focused in this book on providing routines for women trying to conceive, the health and fertility of both partners is, of course, very important. All of the routines we have included in this book would be beneficial for your partner or husband to do as well.

We highly encourage you to practice yoga together as a couple. In addition to improving the health and fertility of both partners, we find that yoga is a great way for couples trying to conceive to "tune-in" to each other. Yoga opens up the energy channels in the body and allows you to be calmer and more present with each other. Doing yoga together is a positive habit to create together. Just like the concept of having an "exercise buddy," it is much easier to keep up your yoga practice if you have a set time of day to practice, and an agreement with your partner to get together at that time to do yoga.

Couples who have been dealing with fertility issues or going through fertility treatments may have discovered that their physical relationship has gotten strained in the process. Being on a schedule for sex, or having to deal with treatment protocols can get in the way of really enjoying each other physically. Doing yoga together is a way to interact in a gentle, physical, non-sexual way without having any of those stresses. Physiologically, practicing yoga together promotes the release of the hormone oxytocin, which is the main human bonding hormone. This is the same hormone that is released during orgasm, and also during breastfeeding.

If you are not able to convince your partner to do the whole routine with you, see if you can at least convince them to do **Legs up the Wall** pose with you, for 5 minutes a day or so. This is a very helpful pose for male fertility, as well. And, they may feel so good after just doing this one pose, that they will be willing to try something else!

7

More Yoga Practices for Fertility Support

Although in the West we may tend to think of yoga as primarily physical postures, yoga as a discipline is much broader than this. Traditional yoga texts talk about the "eight limbs of yoga," with each limb representing a type of practice within the framework of yoga. Physical poses, or asanas, are just one of these eight limbs of yoga. In fact, asanas were traditionally practiced in order to calm the body, increase flexibility and open the energy channels so that the practitioner could sit comfortably for an extended time in meditation.

While it is not within the scope of this book to discuss all of the eight limbs, we would like to offer some practices from a few of these "limbs." The practices

The Eight Limbs of Yoga

Yamas: ethical guidelines on how to act in the world

Niyamas: ethical guidelines on personal behavior and discipline

Asanas: practice of physical poses

Pranayama: conscious breathing practices

Pratyahara: control of the senses, freeing oneself from distraction

Dharana: meditation, concentration, and cultivating self-awareness

Dhyana: devotion; meditation on the Divine

Samadhi: merging of the Self with the Divine

described below are specifically tailored to help reduce stress and enhance fertility. These can be done at the beginning or end of the yoga routines we have offered in earlier chapters, or they can be done as stand-alone practices. You may want to do some of the physical yoga poses first, in order to calm and open the body. This will make sitting still to breathe or meditate easier. You can also do any of the meditations offered below while resting in one of the relaxation poses we have described, such as Legs-up-the-Wall Pose, or supported Cobbler Pose.

CONSCIOUS BREATHING PRACTICE (PRANAYAMA) FOR FERTILITY SUPPORT

Pranayama is simply the practice of breathing consciously. Of course, we breathe all day long without paying the slightest attention to our breath, and without instructing our body to breathe—otherwise we would be able to do nothing else all day long! So, it is possible to have the breath running on "automatic pilot," which we do most of the time. But it is also possible to take conscious control of the breath, and change the way we breathe, which is what we do when we practice pranayama.

Interestingly, breathing is the only bodily function where we can choose to either control it, or put it on auto-pilot. If you want to pick something up, for instance, you will need to consciously think of this, and your brain will need to instruct your hand to do the picking- up action. Other systems, such as the heart, are on auto-pilot, and we don't choose to make it beat or not (although some famous studies conducted at the Menninger Clinic

in the 1970s demonstrated that the accomplished yogi Swami Rama was able to make his heart rate beat 360 beats per minute and then reduce it almost instantly to 52 beats per minute).[1]

Prana, the basis of pranayama, means more than just "breath" in the Western sense of that word. Prana is actually the life-force energy that energizes all aspects of life in the universe. So, when we are breathing, we are bringing in not just oxygen and carbon dioxide, but also life-force energy. With conscious breathing practices, we can bring in more of this life-force energy.

In normal daily breathing, most people use only about 15% of their total breathing capacity, which means that most people are breathing into and out of the upper chest. One of the most basic breathing practices that we do in yoga for fertility is to learn to take the breath all the way into the low belly, thus increasing the quantity of prana we are able to take in on each breath. Also, we can focus the prana into a particular part of the body, if we choose, in order to bring additional life-force energy there. In this case, we are focusing the life-force energy into the low belly area, which contains our center of reproduction.

How to Practice Conscious Breathing for Fertility Support

Yoga breathing is generally done using the nose for both the inhale and exhale. The spine should both lengthen on the inhale and maintain its length during the exhale, without moving the shoulders up and down. *Note: A few specialized breathing practices use the mouth for exhaling, but those practices are not generally* recommended for fertility support. Retaining the breath after inhale is also not recommended for women trying to conceive.

We have offered suggested numbers of rounds for some of the practices. One round is one inhale and one exhale. However, it would be best to do each practice until you have a feeling of calm, even if it takes more than the number of rounds we have suggested.

How to Sit

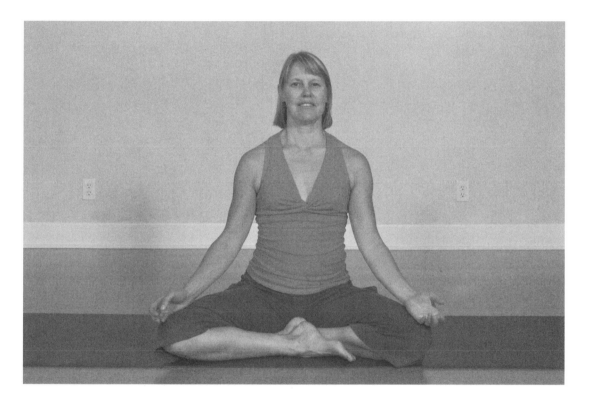

For seated breathing practices, you may want to sit up on the edge of a cushion or blanket to allow hips and knees to open more easily. Seated breathing practice is usually done seated in a comfortable, cross-legged position, in order to keep the lower body grounded and to provide a still and firm base. Start by finding the sitting bones, so that you are sitting straight down through them, not slouching back or leaning forward. Allow the shoulders to relax.

Reach the crown of the head up toward the ceiling. See that your chin is drawn back slightly, and not jutting forward. If the head is pitched forward at all (think of peering at your computer screen, or over the steering wheel of your car), this posture constricts the breath. It is impossible to take long, deep breaths with the chin jutting forward, and yet this is the posture we very commonly see around us, especially in the Western world. *Note: If it is not comfortable for you to sit on the floor, it is also possible to do the breathing practices in a straight-backed chair with a firm seat, maintaining a long spine.*

Effects of Pranayama

Yogic breathing is very calming. All the breathing practices are useful for stress reduction, calming anxiety, reducing insomnia and smoothing out mood swings. From a yoga perspective, this kind of conscious breathing also helps to open the "nadis," which are energy channels that run to all parts of the body.

Pranayama also stimulates the vagus nerve, which is one of the most important nerves in the body, reaching from the brain stem all the way into the belly. This nerve physiologically provides the "plumbing" behind the mind/body connection. Stimulation of the vagus nerve is used by doctors to calm heart palpitations and anxiety, and treat depression, among other things. This effect on the vagus nerve may help explain why pranayama practices are so calming to the central nervous system.

In addition, breathing practices can help with specific things such as:

- balancing the feminine/masculine energy in the body,
- balancing the functions of the sympathetic ("fight-or-flight") and parasympathetic ("relaxation response") nervous systems,
- enhancing the communication between the right hemisphere of the brain (intuitive, creative) and the left (analytical, linear).

YOGA FOR FERTILITY BREATHING PRACTICES

Seated Deep Breathing

Sit in a comfortable seated, cross-legged position. You may want to sit up on one or two folded blankets if your hips, knees or low back are uncomfortable when sitting on the mat without support. Make sure you are sitting straight down on your sitting bones, and the crown of the head is reaching up toward the ceiling. The spine should feel lengthened. Another option is to sit in a chair with a solid seat that will allow you to sit with a long spine. Let your body relax. Begin taking deep, slow inhales and exhales. Try to bring the breath all the way down into the belly on the inhale. Exhale completely. Build in a little pause at the end of the exhale, before you begin inhaling. Do this practice until you begin to feel calm. *Note: for all of these breathing practices, we recommend closing the eyes, if possible, to minimize distractions.*

Ujayii (Audible) Breath

Do the seated deep breathing practice above, but this time try to draw the breath up and down the back of the throat, so that you can hear it moving. You can feel what this is like by opening your mouth and pretending to fog a mirror. Notice the slightly raspy sound and feeling in the back of your throat. Try it on an inhale, by making a gasping noise. Now, see if you can make this sound with the mouth closed. This is what we would like to feel and hear on both the inhale and exhale when we do audible breathing. Try 8–12 rounds.

Belly Breath

Lie on your back with the legs straight, or bend the knees if it is more comfortable for the low back. Take one hand on your belly, the other hand on the low ribcage. Use the hands to feel where your breath is going. Begin by allowing the abdomen to expand on the inhale, then flatten back on the exhale. Try to make the inhale and exhale about the same length, or make the exhale slightly longer. Continue for 12–20 rounds.

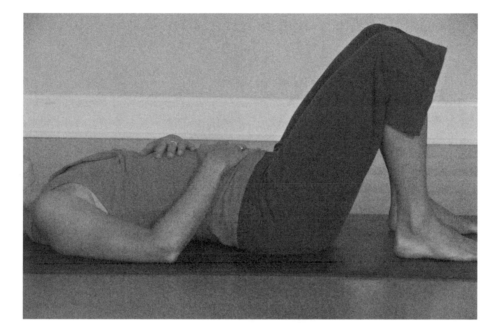

3-Part Abdominal Breathing

After you get comfortable with the Belly Breath, you can try this variation. After expanding the abdomen on the inhale, draw the inhale upwards and expand the ribs, and finally bring the breath all the way up into the chest. Exhale from the top down, starting with the chest, then empty the ribcage, and finally allow the low belly to flatten back toward the spine. Continue for 8–10 rounds.

Counted Breath

Start either sitting comfortably, or lying on the back. Inhale for a slow count of 4, pause slightly, then exhale for a count of 4. Pause after the exhale, before starting the inhale. Repeat. Try 10–12 rounds of this counted breath. Once you are very comfortable with this breath, you can try increasing the count to 6 or 8.

Alternate Nostril Breath

Setup

Sitting comfortably, raise your right hand, and allow your left hand to rest comfortably in your lap. You will be using the thumb and 4th finger (ring finger) of your right hand only. The thumb is used to close the right nostril, and the 4th finger is used for the left.

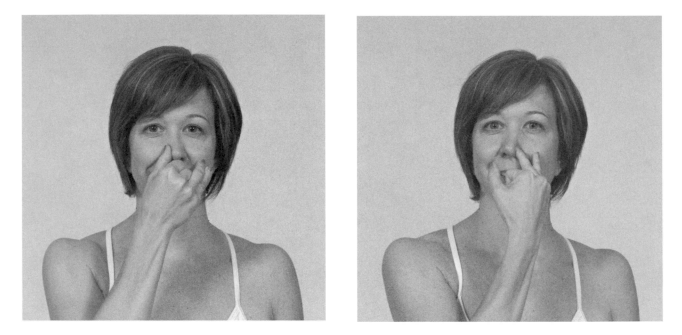

Movement

Begin by exhaling all the air out of the lungs through both nostrils. Close your right nostril with your thumb, and inhale through left nostril only. Pause briefly with the air held in, then close the left nostril using your 4th finger. Exhale through the right nostril only. Make sure to exhale completely. Without moving the hand, and keeping the left nostril closed, inhale through the right nostril only. Using the thumb to close the right nostril, exhale out the left nostril only. Try this for 8 rounds (the whole process described above is one round). You could gradually add more rounds as you become comfortable with this breathing practice.

Why Do This?

Alternate nostril breathing is very calming, and is also useful for balancing the feminine/masculine or yin/yang energy in the body, as well as balancing the left and right brain functions. Breathing through the left nostril activates the right hemisphere of the brain, (the more intuitive, creative side) and breathing through the right nostril activates the left (the more linear, analytical side). In fact, your body automatically does its own alternate nostril breathing, by switching the dominant nostril approximately every 2 ½–4 hours, on a regular schedule!

MEDITATIONS AND VISUALIZATIONS FOR FERTILITY SUPPORT

Meditation is a practice that help focus your attention inwardly, rather than outwardly as we do in normal daily life. Practicing meditation helps develop the capacity to tune out distractions, improving our ability to calm and focus the mind. Meditation can actually be done anywhere, but we recommend trying meditation initially in a quiet environment while seated, or in one of the relaxation postures described in the yoga routine chapters. There are many different ways to do meditation, but they all have similar benefits. We will offer a couple of meditation practices, as well as a few visualization practices specifically for fertility support.

Lucy's Report on Her First Meditation Class

"My mind was wild during my first sit-down meditation. I was thinking about all kinds of things: the Queen of England (?!), why am I here, the cars driving by, etc. The walking meditation worked great for me and I could start to focus and calm my mind down so that when we later went back to seated meditation, I was calm and my brain was settled. The two hours went by in a snap. The teacher said something that was a huge help to me. He said that the goal of meditation is not to block everything out, but to recognize that it is there and basically not let it interfere with our being present. I never knew that, so that alone took a lot of pressure off, and then I could settle into my thoughts without trying too hard to tune out everything else. I just let it be, and then everything was fine."

Meditation can give you a sense of calm and serenity that benefits both your emotional well-being and your overall health. And these benefits don't end when your meditation session ends. Doing a meditation practice in the morning can help you react more calmly to stresses throughout the day. After meditation practice, your body is less likely to go into full "fight-or-flight" mode when your boss finds fault with your project, or your partner criticizes you, or your doctor gives you unwanted news.

Studies have shown that long-term meditators have increased activity in the part of the brain that governs feelings of well-being. Other studies have shown that meditation alters the pattern of brain waves, increasing the presence of calming alpha waves in the brain. "This wave type has been used as a universal sign of relaxation during meditation and other types of rest," comments Professor Øyvind

Benefits of Meditation

- Gaining new perspectives on life situations
- Altering the brain wave pattern which leads to a state of deep relaxation
- Increasing self-awareness
- Noticing negative behavior or thought patterns, and releasing or replacing them
- Disciplining the mind to focus on the present
- Decreasing distractibility
- Reducing negative emotions
- Gaining a general sense of well-being

Ellingsen from the Norwegian University of Science and Technology, one of the lead researchers on a 2010 study of brain wave activity during meditation.[2]

Although there are many different methods of meditating, most of them share some basic elements:

Elements of Meditation

- Choose a quiet environment
- Adopt a comfortable position in which the spine remains lengthened
- Focus attention, for example by "watching" the breath, or through repetition of a word, phrase, prayer or physical activity
- Passive disregard of everyday thoughts
- Non-judgment of any thoughts or feelings that do arise

Following are a couple of basic meditation practices. Some people find it easy to sit and meditate, while others prefer a moving meditation such as mindful walking. You might try the various types to see which approach best helps you to clear the mind and feel calm.

Seated Meditation to Clear the Mind

Setup

Choose a comfortable, seated position where you will be able to sit with a long spine. It is fine to sit on folded blankets or a firm cushion, or with your back against a wall, or even in a straight-backed chair. It is important to be as comfortable as possible to start, so that you are not distracted by aching hips or back during the meditation.

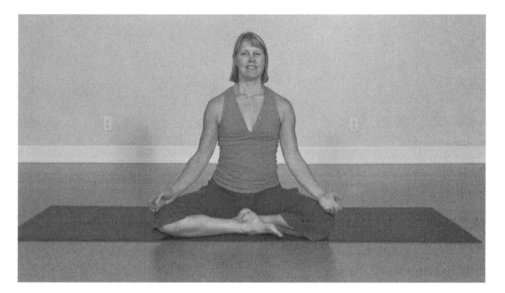

Action

Start by taking several deep, slow breaths to calm the mind. Begin to take your focus to your breath, as you settle into a slow rhythm of breathing. Notice the feeling of the air as it moves into and out of the nostrils. Continue to focus on the breath, without trying to change it. Try to observe any thoughts that come into the mind without following them, getting involved in them, or judging them in any way. Just notice "Oh, there's a thought," and then release it. Be careful not to judge yourself for having thoughts—it is inevitable! In fact, your mind may be going off somewhere every few seconds. The practice is just to notice that, and then bring the focus back to your breath. Try to do this practice for a set amount of time, starting with even just five minutes, and building up as you get more practiced.

Why Do This?

This meditation helps us begin to cultivate an "observer mind," where we can actually stand apart from our thoughts and begin to see patterns of where our mind goes. Often, where it goes is to back to relive negative events or into the future to worry about things. Once we start to notice this, then we can begin to change those patterns, and reroute those thoughts. This is very helpful in reducing stress.

Seated Meditation for Calming

Setup

Choose a comfortable, seated position where you will be able to sit with a long spine. It is fine to sit on folded blankets or a firm cushion, or with your back against a wall, or even in a straight-backed chair. It is important to be as comfortable as possible to start, so that you are not distracted by aching hips or back during the meditation.

Action

This meditation uses the technique of repeating a word or phrase as a focal point. Choose words or phrases that feel calming and soothing to you. For example, you could choose the words "calm," and "peace," or the phrases "I am calm" and "I am peaceful." Start by taking several deep, slow breaths. Then begin to mentally repeat the word(s), tying the words to the breath. As you inhale, mentally say the words "I am calm," and as you exhale, say the words "I am peaceful." Try to do this practice for a set amount of time, starting with just a few minutes, and adding time as you get more practiced.

Why Do This?

The messages we give ourselves about events are important in determining our body's reactions to those events. This meditation helps us learn to change the way we feel by changing our thoughts.

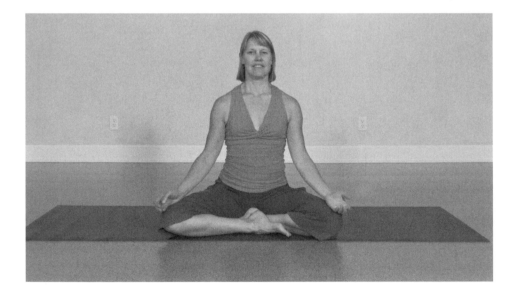

Mindful Walking Meditation

Setup

This is a moving meditation practicing "mindfulness." Choose a location where you will be able to walk in natural surroundings, without traffic, such as a park, or a beach. Wear comfortable walking shoes, and dress for the weather. You may want to choose a route that is a short loop, or a path that you can follow for a short way out and back.

Action

Start by standing in one place, and looking around you. Notice the colors you see: in the sky, the trees, the water. Notice any nature sounds: birds singing, leaves rustling, water splashing. Notice any smells: a flowering tree, salt air. Notice any sensations: the feel of a breeze in your hair, the rocks underfoot. Pay attention to any details that catch your eye, and really take a moment to *see* them: drops of dew on the grass, a beautiful rock, a spider's web. Begin walking slowly, continuing to notice and take in what is around you, staying present with where you are. If your mind strays off to some thought that has nothing to do with where you are, just notice that, and gently bring your attention back to noticing what is around you.

Why Do This?

This meditation helps us learn to stay present, and really notice the beauty of the world around us. Often, we are so absorbed in our thoughts that we are living totally in our heads. Being absorbed in our own thoughts may mean we are stuck in negative loops, or worrying all the time. Learning to stay present gives us a break from these thoughts, and reintroduces us to the beauty of nature. It is amazing how good such a simple practice can make us feel!

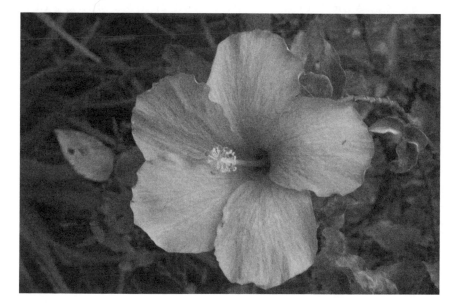

Passage Meditation

Setup

This practice can be done in a comfortable seated position or lying on your back.

Action

Find a passage of a prayer or spiritual teaching that resonates with you. Print out the passage or write it down on a piece of paper and have it close by when you are ready to begin. At first, you may have to read the passage with your eyes open before you memorize it. Keep reading or repeating the passage in your mind over and over again. You can try to do this meditation for 5 or 10 minutes at first, eventually building up to 30 minutes. It will probably not take you very long to memorize the passage and you can take away the printed version when you no longer need it and practice this meditation with the eyes closed. What may be more challenging, is keeping your mind on the passage without it wandering off to other more exciting things. When you notice your mind wandering away from the passage, simply acknowledge that and come back to the repetition of the passage. If you don't remember where you left off, simply go back to beginning and keep repeating the passage.

Why Do This?

Passage meditation was developed by Eknath Easwaran as part of the Eight Point Program outlined in his book "Passage Meditation." The idea of repeating an inspirational passage is to help you to focus your mind on something deeper than surface thoughts. The hope is that these inspirational words will eventually make their way into your subconscious to create meaningful change in your life. It has the same benefits of the other types of meditation and can be especially helpful if you are having trouble slowing down your thoughts during meditation, or would like to change a pattern of thinking or behaving.

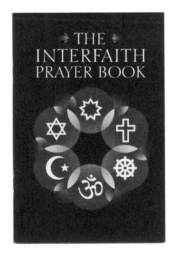

Heart-to-Uterus Visualization

Setup

For this practice, you could sit comfortably, or lie on your back. It is also a good practice to combine with legs-up-the-wall pose.

Action

Begin by taking a few deep inhales and exhales. Take your focus to the center of your heart, and imagine that with each breath, you are inhaling into the heart center, and exhaling out of the heart center. Now, begin to imagine that as you inhale into the heart, you also draw the breath from the heart down to the low belly area. If you are able to visualize drawing it directly into the uterus, you could do that. On the exhale, allow any tension or holding to release out of the pelvic area. With each breath, feel that you are drawing heart energy down to the low belly, and infusing your reproductive organs with this positive heart energy. If you like, you can visualize the heart energy as warm, green light, flowing with the inhale down into the low belly/pelvic bowl, and surrounding the uterus and ovaries with this green light. You could also choose one of the positive attributes of heart energy to focus on, such as love, compassion, forgiveness, nurture, joy or hope.

Why Do This?

In yoga, we consider the heart area to be a key energy center, and the pelvic area to be another key energy center. The energy of the heart center contains positive, nurturing, loving energy. Chinese medicine recognizes a meridian, or energy channel, which runs from the heart to the uterus, and explains that this heart-to-uterus energy channel needs to be open in order for conception to occur.

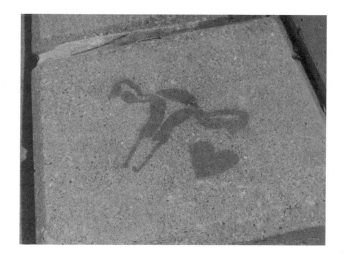

AFFIRMATIONS FOR FERTILITY SUPPORT

The more we learn about the mind/body connection, the more clear it becomes that the body really does physically react to the messages it is receiving from the mind, whether these messages are conscious or not. Dr. Christiane Northrup is well known for working with women's health issues from both a physical and an emotional/mental perspective. She says, "Mental and emotional energy goes in and out of physical form regularly. . . . Quite simply, emotional and mental energy can become physical in our bodies."[3] Likewise, in his book *The Mind-Body Fertility Connection*, James Schwarz says, "When a negative emotional signal is communicated to the physical body, it can cause a block or disturbance in the flow of healthy chi which, in turn, can create a physical disharmony."[4]

When facing fertility challenges, an underlying problem may be that we are sending ourselves messages that are affecting our physical body in a way that is not supportive of ovulation or conception. These messages could be conscious, but more likely these are subconscious messages that may, on the face of it, have nothing to do with fertility. How important are subconscious messages? An article published in *U.S. News and World Report* in 2005 states, "According to cognitive neuroscientists, we are conscious of only about 5 percent of our cognitive activity, so most of our decisions, actions, emotions and behavior depend on the 95 percent of brain activity that goes beyond our conscious awareness."[5]

Notice that fear figures prominently in many negative subconscious messages. These messages most likely got implanted in childhood, and so have had many years to get embedded in our psyches. Overcoming these is not a simple matter, but we can start by trying to see what they are—in other words, allowing ourselves to feel them honestly. Often we have tried for so long to bury these messages, that we fear even allowing ourselves to accept that they exist. Once we do, we can practice replacing them with messages that emphasize faith, rather than fear. We call these positive messages "affirmations."

Subconscious Messages that May Affect Fertility

"I am not adequate" (which may actually mean "I am not perfect")

"I might lose control" (fear of looking foolish, or doing something I will regret)

"I will be abandoned" (fear of loss, fear of being left alone)

"I won't get the support I need" (fear of having to do everything myself)

Using Affirmations

Since we are trying to change negative thought and energy patterns with our affirmations, it is important to practice these regularly. Setting aside a few minutes to focus on your affirmations a few times a day is one way to do this. You could also write the affirmations on sticky notes and post them in places where you will be sure to see them during the day, such as on your computer screen, on the refrigerator door, or on the dashboard of your car. You can use any affirmations that appeal to you, or write your own. It is very important that the affirmations be stated in the present tense, not in the future. It may be worthwhile to "try on" the affirmations on our list, one at a time, and note any that make you feel particularly uncomfortable when you say them. If an affirmation makes you particularly uncomfortable, this probably means that there is a strong subconscious message telling you that the opposite is true.

Fertility Affirmations

I am fertile.

I will conceive.

I am taking charge of my fertility.

I am healthy and whole and full of love.

I am blessed.

I am thankful for all that I am and all that I have. I am at peace.

My eggs are healthy and happy.

I will hold my baby in my arms.

I am beautiful and healthy, and so is my baby.

I am open to the energy of birth.

Our healthy, happy baby will arrive at the perfect time.

Some of the most impressive success stories from my yoga for fertility classes have been from women who made strong use of affirmations. It is an extremely powerful practice. Affirmations can also be used when some "fertility expert" says that there is a small chance, or even no chance, of conceiving. In this case, the affirmations are helping to overcome not only subconscious messaging, but messages from external "experts." Over the years, several women in my classes have successfully conceived after being told their chances were something like ".05%." These women used a combination of approaches, with positive affirmations being a key component.

VISION BOARDS AND FERTILITY "ALTARS"

One of my favorite authors is Dr. Deepak Chopra, a kind of modern-day guru who is a medical doctor as well as a prolific writer. Dr. Chopra has an astonishing ability to explain complex Eastern philosophical concepts to Westerners in simple language. One of my favorite concepts he offers is: "What you focus on expands in your life." This is a great condensation of one of the basic principles of the universe, according to yogic philosophy—that *action follows energy*. This principle shows why it is so important for us to pay attention to what thoughts we allow to fill our minds. The outcome of a situation (action) will be determined by where and how energy is directed in that situation.

Some of the techniques that have been used by my students to keep their energy focused on positive outcomes include vision boards and fertility "altars."

A vision board can be as simple as a sheet of poster board or cardboard, covered with photographs cut from magazines. One of my students did a high-tech version that she used as a screen-saver on her computer. The idea is to include any images or words that represent fertility to you. They could be obvious ones, such as photos of babies or pregnant women, or more symbolic, such as blooming flowers or green fields. This is very personal and individual, so include images that are meaningful to you. Then, post your vision board in a prominent place where you will see it several times a day.

A fertility "altar" is another way to keep your fertility focus on the positive. It is basically a "3-D" vision board, where you set aside a small space in your home to place any objects or images that represent fertility to you. These could include flowers, books, photos, rocks or gems, carvings, candles, jewelry, baby shoes—anything that represents your vision of your pregnancy and/or your baby. One of my students made a small fertility altar on her bedside stand, so that she saw it just before she went to sleep and as soon as she woke up. Other students have had fertility talismans that they carried or wore during the day. One woman had a heart-shaped rock that represented her heart connection to her baby. Another wore a necklace that said "miracles happen every day." This woman had been told by every fertility clinic in her city that her only chance to conceive was via donor egg; she went on to "miraculously" conceive two children with her own eggs.

CHANTING

Chanting involves either repeating a word or phrase out loud, or singing words or phrases. The vocalizing is important, and distinguishes chanting from meditating, where we may be repeating words or phrases mentally. As with the breathing practices, chanting also stimulates the vagus nerve. This is effected through muscle movements in the mouth, as well as vibrations of the vocal chords. Thus, the act of chanting can be very relaxing to the central nervous system. There are other powerful reasons to add chanting to your fertility "toolkit."

Chanting has a strong relationship to fertility due to the relationships between the main energy centers in the body, the chakras. The energy center in the throat (throat chakra) is partnered with the reproductive energy center (sacral chakra) in the low belly. So, any practices we can do that help to open the throat chakra, also help to open and release tension in the reproductive center.

Another reason for incorporating chanting into your fertility practices is simply the power of the chants themselves. In the yogic tradition, there are key words or phrases, called mantras, which are believed to hold special power to transform consciousness, promote healing, or fulfill desires. Chanting these mantras, even if you didn't know the meaning of them, would invoke the power invested in the mantra.

How to Chant

Sit in a comfortable seated position, as for breathing practice, with a lengthened spine. Sitting up on cushions or sitting in a straight-backed chair is fine. Rest the hands on the knees. If you rest the hands palms up, you will be receiving extra energy from the chanting through the palms of the hands. Now, choose one of the following chants to repeat. You could just repeat the chant in a single tone, or you could add a simple tune to the words. Traditionally, yogis count the mantras using a loop of 108 beads, called mala beads. However, you could count repetitions on your fingers, or just repeat the mantras without counting. There are certain numbers of repetitions that are considered to be most powerful, including 108, and 54. But any chanting you do will be powerful. Below are some suggested chants that are appropriate for fertility. These are in Sanskrit, the ancient language of yoga, and we have tried to supply an approximate pronunciation and interpretation for these. You could also use any of your affirmations as chants, by repeating them out loud, or setting them to a tune, or choose a single word such as "peace", "calm", or "acceptance".

Chants to Support Fertility

OM (pronounced with a long "O") This chant brings you in tune with the underlying current of creative energy that sustains the universe.

OM Kleem (pronounced like "clean" with an "m" at the end) This chant is a request that all your desires be fulfilled.

OM Gung Ganapataye Namah (Om gung gone-ah-pot–ah-yay na-ma) This chant is used to help remove obstacles in our paths.

OM Sri Dhanvantariye Namah (Om shri don-von-taree-yay na-ma) This chant asks for healing, and to restore health.

8

Lifestyle Changes to Support Fertility

"Lifestyle" is a broad term, and includes many components which can impact fertility. We have chosen several areas to address in this chapter, based on the areas that we have most often observed to be impacting fertility in our students. In selecting these areas to address, we have also considered the degree to which one is able to make changes in them. To begin with, there is a fair amount of controversy regarding how these "lifestyle" components affect fertility. While some research has been done, much more is needed to round out our knowledge of the optimal approach to take from a fertility standpoint. Our recommendations are based on our training, consultations with various types of practitioners who work with fertility issues, observations of our students over the years, review of the existing research, and our own personal experience.

FERTILITY NUTRITION

It is possible to find contradictory advice by just a cursory review of published information on the subject of nutrition and fertility. Several distinct approaches to fertility nutrition exist. Among these approaches, some recommendations are fairly universal, and then there are some that are in conflict with each other.

DIFFERENT APPROACHES TO FERTILITY NUTRITION

■ the Traditional Chinese Medicine approach,
■ the approach taken by Western-trained dieticians,
■ the food sensitivities approach,
■ the Ayurvedic approach,
■ the "whole foods" approach.

You may want to decide which approach you want to follow, in order to simplify this question of fertility nutrition enough to apply it to your life. We have seen good results with all of these approaches. However, it is important to work with a practitioner who understands the approach you have chosen and can coach you with this process. Following is a very basic description of each of the above-listed approaches to fertility nutrition.

THE TRADITIONAL CHINESE MEDICINE APPROACH

If you are working with a doctor of Oriental medicine or an acupuncturist, it is likely that they will give you nutritional recommendations based on your Chinese medicine diagnosis. For example, if she or he diagnoses kidney Yin deficiency, your doctor or acupuncturist may give you a list of foods that help build kidney Yin. Beyond this, there are some general recommendations that are common in Chinese medicine. For example, dairy products are generally considered unhelpful for fertility, although red meat is sometimes recommended, depending on your diagnosis. A good discussion of fertility nutrition recommendations from the Chinese medicine perspective is included in the book *The Infertility Cure*, by Dr. Randine Lewis.

THE WESTERN DIETICIAN APPROACH

You will get "Western" nutritional advice if you decide to see an R.D. (registered dietician). The general focus of this kind of nutritional advice is to eat a balanced diet with plenty of fiber, fruits and vegetables. Dairy and meat are not normally restricted on this type of diet. Recommendations may be made for reduced intake of fats, especially partially hydrogenated fats, sugar and processed foods. Many women seeking pregnancies have improved their diet and nutrition by following this approach.

Interestingly, one recommendation that we have heard is that full-fat dairy products are more supportive of fertility than nonfat or low-fat. This recommendation is based on the data gathered in the Nurses' Study, a long-term study which has been following a large group of women over a period of over twenty years. The study results showed that the women ingesting nonfat or low-fat dairy products had increased incidences of anovulatory infertility. In contrast, ingesting full-fat dairy products, including milk and ice cream, appeared to reduce the incidence of anovulatory infertility. [1]

THE FOOD SENSITIVITIES APPROACH

Doctors of Naturopathy often consider food sensitivities in recommending a fertility diet. The general concept is that some people, while not having actual food allergies, may have a heightened sensitivity to certain foods or food groups. Although the reaction to these foods will not be life-threatening, it can cause lower-level reactions leading to systemic inflammation. It is believed that inflammation in the body can inhibit implantation, and may also interfere with ovulation. Food sensitivity diets are usually very individualized. Common foods that may cause food sensitivity leading to inflammation include wheat, dairy, soy, corn and gluten.

Our observation has been that students who have had food sensitivities identified, and who have modified their diets to eliminate these foods, have noticed a general improvement in health. For example, one of my students who was about to start an IVF cycle decided to try eliminating gluten, although she was very skeptical. When she came back to see me 3 weeks later she told me that the first few days after she took gluten out of her diet she had so much energy she couldn't sleep! After that, her sleep returned to normal, but she noticed that her general energy level was much higher than before. She was thrilled to have discovered this, and planned to continue on her gluten-free diet.

THE AYURVEDIC APPROACH

Ayurveda is the "medical" branch of yoga, which has been practiced in India and surrounding areas for thousands of years. Many people consider Ayurveda to be the oldest body of medical knowledge. Ayurvedic dietary recommendations are based on a person's constitutional type, or prakriti, which is the initial assessment an Ayurvedic physician will make. From a fertility perspective, certain foods and herbs are considered to boost fertility, and there may be different recommendations for female fertility versus male fertility. Our observations have been that eating a diet based on Ayurvedic principles can be very helpful in achieving an overall life balance, and also can boost fertility.

THE WHOLE FOODS APPROACH

The "whole foods" approach to fertility nutrition tends to recommend limiting animal-based products, and replacing them with plant-based proteins such as soy, legumes, nuts or grains. There is also an emphasis on fresh fruits and vegetables. Common restrictions include: processed foods, white flour, sugar and sometimes meat and dairy products. Fats should be "good" fats, such as olive oil or coconut oil, not butter or partially hydrogenated fats. A good resource book for a fertility diet based on the whole foods approach is *Cooking for Fertility* by Kathryn Simmons Flynn.

To help sort all of this out, below is an overview of our general recommendations for eating for optimal fertility:

OUR TOP 15 RECOMMENDATIONS FOR FERTILITY NUTRITION

Increase

1. Increase your intake of vegetables of all colors. Include plenty of dark green leafy vegetables like kale, Swiss chard, spinach (cooked, not raw), dark or colored lettuces (not Iceberg). Lightly cooked vegetables are preferable to raw.

2. Replace white flour with whole grains such as oats, barley, and quinoa; Since wheat is one of the common food sensitivities, try to choose other grains such as

(continued)

spelt or rice for breads and pastas. Buckwheat is not, in fact, a type of wheat, so this is also a good choice. Most of the corn used in the U.S. is genetically modified, so if you choose corn products, make sure they are organic.

3. Choose organic fruits and vegetables whenever possible. Some types of fruits and veggies are more pesticide-intensive to grow, so it is particularly important to choose organic for these. Limit citrus fruits and juices, as these can contribute to an acidic environment in the body. Acidic cervical mucus is hostile to sperm.

4. Increase sources of Omega3 fatty acids, such as salmon, tuna, mackerel, if you eat meat. However, limit consumption of tuna to twice a week, due to concerns about mercury build-up in these fish. Walnuts, hemp products, blue-green algae and flax seed are vegetarian sources

5. Ensure adequate intake of folic acid (at least 700 mcg/day) from plant sources or supplements. Good food sources include: legumes, dark leafy green vegetables, oranges, yams, cantaloupes and fortified grains or cereals.

6. Get 40–80 mcg/day of nonheme (from plant sources) iron. Good sources are: pumpkin seeds, spinach, dried fruit, kidney beans, nuts, acorn squash, and enriched breads, cereals or rice.

7. Take supplemental Vitamin D if you live in an area that does not have sunny weather all year, especially if you limit dairy consumption. You should have at least 1,000-2,000 IU's/day. Vitamin D is thought to play a role in egg formation. Also include choline in your diet; eggs are a good source.

8. Drink plenty of room temperature water, or hot tea. Iced beverages disrupt the digestive process, so avoid these. Invest in a countertop water filter if you don't have one. Avoid buying water in plastic bottles at the store, due to possible endocrine-inhibitors in the plastic.

Limit

9. Eliminate sodas, both regular and diet. These contain either way too much sugar, or chemicals to replace the sugar. Artificial sweeteners such as aspartame may disrupt the pituitary function, which in turn impacts the ovaries.

10. Reduce caffeine intake. Switch from coffee to green tea. Some Chinese practitioners feel that the toxins in coffee are even worse than the caffeine, so they may also recommend eliminating decaf coffee when trying to conceive. (Note that the Nurse's Study showed no effect of moderate caffeine intake on fertility).[2]

11. Eliminate partially hydrogenated fats, which have been linked to inflammation in the body. Be careful—many packaged and processed foods contain these!

12. Restrict intake of sugar and white flour. Some practitioners believe that everyone has a food sensitivity to white sugar; i.e., that it produces inflammation in everyone's bodies.

13. If using dairy, choose full-fat, organic products. Non-organic dairy can contain extra estrogen from the hormones given the cows to increase milk production. Plain yogurt would be the best dairy choice, since many people with dairy sensitivity can still tolerate yogurt. Yogurt also contains probiotics, which bolster the immune system.

14. If eating meat, choose organic meats to avoid added hormones and antibiotics. This is most important with red meats and pork.
15. Reduce or eliminate alcohol intake. Alcohol impacts the liver, and the liver is responsible for removing excess hormones from the bloodstream. Some studies have found decreased fertility from even modest alcohol consumption. (Note that the Nurse's Study found no effect of moderate consumption, equal to about one 5 oz. glass of wine per day).[3]

It is a good idea is to wash all fruits and vegetables, whether or not they are organic, with a food-grade detergent. You can order this type of product at http://www.environne.com. A list of the most important fruits and veggies to buy organically can be found at: www.foodnews.org.

MINDFUL EATING

In addition to choosing the right foods, the nutritional value of food is also affected by how you eat, and how you prepare the food. Here are some suggestions to increase the benefit you receive from the food you eat:

Eating to Increase Nutritional Value of Food

- When you are cooking, pay attention to the preparation, and mindfully focus your positive energy on the task. If you are in a bad mood when you cook, that energy goes into the food.
- Before you eat, take a moment to feel gratitude for the people that prepared it (even if it was you!) and the farmers that grew it.
- Turn off the TV, and especially avoid watching the news during meals. Taking in negative energy while you are eating negatively impacts digestion, and your ability to make use of the nutrients.
- Try eating without multi-tasking, but just focusing on the food. You will eat more slowly, notice the flavors more, enjoy your meal more, and get more nutritional value, too!

NUTRITIONAL DEFICIENCIES

This is another area that is ripe with controversy; however, we have observed that supplementation of certain nutrients has, in some cases, resulted in pregnancies carried to term where this was not possible before. While a major deficiency in any of the key vitamins or minerals can almost certainly impact fertility, such deficiencies are not that common in the United States. Instead, we will focus on a few nutritional deficiencies that are potentially common, and perhaps not normally considered in a fertility workup. Deficiencies in these nutrients are considered by some practitioners to have an adverse affect on fertility.

Vitamin D3

Vitamin D3 is one of the most common vitamins which requires supplementation. Since the most common source of vitamin D is sunlight, areas of the country where winters are long and cloudy (like where I live in Seattle!) don't provide enough sunlight to meet the body's needs. The other major source of vitamin D3 is dairy products, which have vitamin D added. As more women eliminate dairy from their diets, this source of D3 has been impacted. Dairy replacements, such as soy, rice or almond milk, also have added vitamin D. However it is in the form of D2, which is not as easily absorbed by the body as D3, which is added to dairy.

Low vitamin D is implicated in many conditions, including reduced fertility, depression, and poor immune system function. Most naturopaths routinely check vitamin D levels, and most clinics will test if you ask them to. Supplementation is simple, and involves taking a few drops of a vitamin D suspension, or tablets. If the blood level of vitamin D is very low, your doctor may recommend several thousand IU's per day for several weeks, in order to bring the level up relatively quickly. However, as vitamin D can be toxic in excess, you should work with a physician who can test and monitor your levels. It is not possible to take in excess amounts of vitamin D from the sun—only from supplements.

Vitamin B12

Vitamin B12 not only helps your body to produce red blood cells, it also helps keep your nervous system healthy. Vitamin B12 deficiencies have been linked to reduced fertility. Although severe Vitamin B12 deficiency is rare, certain conditions make it more likely. Vitamin B12 is present in meat, eggs and dairy products, so people following a strict vegan diet tend to be more at risk of developing a vitamin B12 deficiency. However, it can also be found in some vegan foods, such as fortified cereals and soy products. Nutritional yeast is a very good source.

Vitamin B12 has a complex way of being absorbed by the stomach and small intestine, so procedures which interfere with those areas, such as gastric bypass surgery, may make vitamin B12 deficiency more likely. Other conditions which may impact Vitamin B12 absorbtion include celiac disease, Crohn's disease and HIV. Most naturopathic physicians will test B12 levels, and most other clinics will do so if you request it.

MTHFR

MTHFR, or methylene tetrahydrofolate reductase, is an enzyme responsible for folate metabolism in the body. This enzyme converts the folate/folic acid we eat (or take as supplements) into methylfolate, which is the usable form for our bodies. In some individuals there is a genetic mutation, or marker, which causes the enzyme to not be fully functioning.

The two most common mutations are known as C677T and A1298C. An individual can have one or both copies of these. MTHFR has links to many diseases in the scientific literature, including depression, migraines, cancer, birth defects and recurrent miscarriages. It is commonly checked in women trying to get pregnant if a clotting abnormality is suspected. Otherwise, it is not generally tested for in fertility clinics or by OB/Gyns; however, most clinics will test for the MTHFR markers if you request it.

A person with one or both genetic markers could be taking a lot of folic acid, but still have very low levels of folic acid in their system. Just taking additional folic acid supplements will not help, because their body is unable to convert folic acid into a usable form. Folic acid is a crucial nutrient, especially for pregnant women.

Low levels of folic acid can contribute to serious birth defects of the brain and spinal cord. Folic acid levels must be adequate during pre-conception, as well as in the early weeks of pregnancy, in order to avoid these neural tube defects.

Treatment for the MTHFR defect is relatively simple, and includes taking L-methylfolate as a supplement, rather than taking a supplement with regular folic acid. L-Methyl Folate is now available in the appropriate dose without a prescription. It is sold as 5-MTHF by several companies including Thorne and Metabolic Maintenance and the appropriate dose is 5–10 mg.

There is much remaining to be learned about the effects of MTHFR on fertility, and large studies are needed. If you have tested positive for one or both genetic markers, it is important to find an allopathic or naturopathic physician familiar with the disorder, as this needs to be treated prior to attempting to conceive. If you have personal or family history of miscarriage, it would be worthwhile to be tested for these markers. However, other issues can cause miscarriage, so it would be important to consult a physician specializing in fertility to test for other factors, as well.

WEIGHT AND FERTILITY

There is a general consensus that an optimal range of BMIs (Body Mass Index) exist for fertility. Body Mass is calculated by a ratio of height versus weight. If your weight falls either above or below the optimal range, your weight may be impacting your ability to get pregnant. Either a high or a low BMI can impact hormonal levels in the body. Since body fat contains estrogen receptors, women with high BMIs often have excess estrogen, and women with low BMIs may have low estrogen levels. Below is a chart showing normal BMI levels, and levels considered above normal.[4] Anything below a 19 BMI is considered underweight. You can see where you fall in the BMI chart by finding your height on the left-hand column, and your weight in the chart. The optimal range for fertility is the "Normal" range, a BMI of between 19–24.

	Normal	Overweight	Obese	Extreme Obesity
	BMI 19–24	BMI 25–29	BMI 30–35	BMI 40–54
5'0"	93–123 lbs	128–149 lbs	154–200 lbs	205–277 lbs
5'3"	107–135 lbs	141–183 lbs	189–220 lbs	225–304 lbs
5'7"	121–153 lbs	159–185 lbs	191–249 lbs	255–314 lbs
5'10"	133–167 lbs	174–202 lbs	217–272 lbs	279–377 lbs

You can also determine your own BMI using the online BMI calculator at: www.nhlbisupport.com/bmi or http://www.conceiveonline.com/content/bmi-calculator.

If you are under the normal BMI range, simply gaining enough weight to put you back in the "normal" range can boost fertility considerably. If you are above the normal BMI range, consider a combination of diet and exercise. However, weight loss should be gradual, as precipitous weight loss can also adversely affect fertility.

EXERCISE

The impact of exercise on fertility is another area that has been rife with conflicting opinions and advice. For many years, fertility clinics were telling their patients that they could continue to do any exercise that they were used to doing, but not to start up new exercise programs while trying to conceive (unless it was specifically for weight loss due to a high BMI). Based on the outcome of some recent studies, however, the advice is beginning to change. Studies have recently shown that while moderate exercise such as walking, yoga, and gardening may benefit fertility, more vigorous exercise may negatively impact fertility.

A study, completed in 2006 and funded by the National Institute of Health, looked at IVF outcomes relative to levels of exercise.[6] This study showed that women who reported exercising at least 4 hours per week for one to nine years prior to their IVF cycle were 40% less likely to have a live birth than women who reported no exercise. The study was particularly thorough, in that it looked at exercise patterns for the years leading up to the IVF cycle, not just exercise immediately prior to or during the cycle. "Regular exercise before

Vigorous Exercise Delays Pregnancy in Normal-Weight Women

A recent study by Danish and US researchers found that vigorous exercise led to longer times to conception in healthy, normal- weight women (BMI under 25). In overweight and obese women (BMI above 25) vigorous physical activity did not result in delays.

Activities such as running, fast cycling, aerobics, gymnastics, and swimming were characterized as vigorous. Brisk walking, leisurely cycling, golfing and gardening were considered moderate. Moderate physical activity was associated with improved time to pregnancy across the range of BMI.

Linda Giudice, MD, PhD, noted, "This study is particularly interesting because its participants were recruited from the general population, not from infertility patients. It points out the benefits of moderate exercise to all women who are planning a pregnancy and suggests that women might reduce their time to pregnancy by modulating their exercise programs."[5]

in vitro fertilization may negatively affect outcomes, especially in women who exercised four or more hours per week for 1–9 years, and those who participated in cardiovascular exercise," according to the study authors. An interesting note is that women who had exercised for longer than 9 years showed no negative impact on IVF outcome. One theory is that, after exercising for such a long time, their bodies had adjusted to the exercise as "normal," rather than as a stressor.

Finally, we would like to mention a study that looked at the impact of a combination of exercise, dieting and stress on fertility.[7] This study was carried out on monkeys, but the implications for female humans are worth noting. The study was particularly interesting because the impact of each of the three factors was studied separately, and then in combination. When the monkeys were subjected to either mild stress, *or* restricted-calorie diets, *or* an exercise program, ten percent of the monkeys stopped having periods. However, when the monkeys were subjected to stress *as well as* restricted diet and exercise, *seventy-five percent* stopped having periods. If these results can be extrapolated to human females who are trying to conceive, and who are likely under some amount of stress, then adding exercise and/or dieting may have a very negative effect on fertility.

What we have been recommending to our yoga for fertility students for years regarding exercise is that vigorous exercise is not helpful when trying to conceive. I can personally say that I have never had a student fail to get pregnant because she was "out of shape," unless the student was in a very high BMI category, and really needed to lose weight. I have had a number of students fail to get pregnant, in my opinion, because they refused to stop going to the gym and doing their daily workouts. And, I have had a number of students who became pregnant, after several years of trying, when a move or an injury or other life event disrupted the exercise program they had been following.

At least in Seattle, suggesting that someone back off their exercise program is rarely a popular suggestion. Some women have actually decided to *start* a new exercise program with the idea that they need to "get healthy" so that they can get pregnant. And it seems all of our lives we have heard that exercising is healthy, so this advice may seem counterintuitive. As noted in the studies cited above, although there is more and more evidence that this is the case, there is not yet a clear understanding as to why more strenuous exercise appears to have a negative impact on fertility. Some theories include:

Some Theories on Why Exercise May Negatively Affect Fertility

- The authors of the IVF and exercise study suggest that it may have to do with the impact on hormone levels: "Intense aerobic exercise may inhibit release of gonadotropin-releasing hormone and result in a hypoestrogenic state, while women who perform heavy resistance training may increase levels of luteinizing hormone and androgen. Leptin and insulin levels may decrease with intense exercise."[8]
- Dr. Alice Domar suggests that, "Progesterone production might be adversely affected by exercise, thus preventing embryo implantation."[9]
- Some researchers have theorized that exercise disrupts the communication between the hypothalamus and the pituitary gland, thus impacting the production and release of reproductive hormones such as LH and FSH.[10]

Our recommendation for a good fertility-supporting exercise program is to do a daily practice of yoga for fertility and walk (outdoors, if possible). If you are a golfer, or a gardener, or enjoy leisurely cycling, you may also include these instead of, or in addition to, walking, since they are gentle and also take place outdoors. We feel that exercising outdoors has multiple benefits and so we recommend walking outdoors as opposed to walking on a treadmill, if the weather permits. Studies have shown that being out in nature is calming to the mind and the central nervous system, so walking in a park, or just in a neighborhood with trees, grass or flowers can be stress-reducing. Also, being exposed to natural light helps regulate the body's cycles and rhythms, including the reproductive cycle. Dr. Christiane Northrup says, "Living in artificial light without going outside into natural sunlight regularly can have adverse consequences on fertility, because light itself is a nutrient."[11]

On Using Exercise for Stress Reduction

One argument I regularly hear from students is that their current exercise program is crucial because it helps them deal with the stress in their lives, and without it, they will be more stressed, which isn't good for fertility. My usual response to this is offering them what I call my "two-week challenge." I suggest that they take just two weeks to try doing a daily yoga for fertility practice, and take a daily walk, instead of the hour they usually spend at the gym, or out running. If at the end of two weeks, they are still feeling the need to do their vigorous exercise program for stress reduction, they should come back and tell me, and we will negotiate. In the ten years I have been making this recommendation, *no one* has ever come back and said they still needed their vigorous exercise program. In fact, some women have come back and said they didn't realize how draining their exercise program was until they replaced it with these gentler, but still stress-reducing, practices.

We have been recommending a less-strenuous exercise program when trying to conceive, even prior to the recent Western scientific studies on this topic. From our yoga training, and also from Chinese medicine theories, we understand that people have a certain amount of internal "essence" to draw from. If we are working in a stressful job, or have other life stresses, this uses up our "essence." If on top of that, we are doing vigorous exercise which also uses "essence," we end up with a deficit. Over time, continuing to do these activities which cost us "essence" lowers our immunity and our vitality, including our reproductive vitality. Instead, we need to do activities such as gentle yoga and walking in nature, which replenish our "essence," to offset other parts of our lives where we may be using it up. This is always important, but even more so if you are trying to conceive.

In Chinese medicine, this "essence" is called "Jing." An excellent description of this concept of "essence," or "Jing," is provided by Dr. Jeanie Lee Bussell:

> *Jing is your "Youthful Essence," but also your reproductive essence. When we are born, we are full of Jing. But as we live and age, we consume it. This is similar to how a candle must burn its wax in order to give light. Everyone uses up their Jing at different rates. Some deplete their Jing much faster than others; especially those whose lifestyle, diet and attitudes are out of balance. . . Lack of Jing can sometimes be seen as premature signs of aging: premature graying of the hair, wrinkles, and diminished reproductive capacity. On a daily basis, Jing can be acquired through diet, and through exercise such as Qi Gong. But if you burn through your Jing faster than you can acquire it, you will speed your aging and impair your body's functioning.* [12]

WORK AND RELATIONSHIPS

This concept of "essence" can be applied to other areas of your life, in addition to exercise. For example, your work can be adding to your essence, if it is work that is fulfilling for you. Or, it can be draining your essence if it is stressful and you don't get much joy out of it. If it is draining, is it possible to change your situation so that it is more fulfilling, or change your hours so that it is less draining? You can put the relationships in your life to the same test: are they replenishing your essence, or are they draining it? If you find that you are in relationships that are draining rather than fulfilling, can you make changes that either help them be more fulfilling, or limit the time you spend with people that are draining you?

Top Five Lifestyle Changes for Fertility: Our Recommendations

1. Follow our Top 15 Recommendations for Fertility Nutrition set out earlier in this chapter.
2. Keep a regular (early) bedtime, and get plenty of sleep.
3. If you aren't exercising, or if you have been doing a vigorous exercise program, try daily yoga and walking instead.
4. Look at your work and relationships from the perspective of whether they are building essence, or draining it. Make changes as you can.
5. Let go and accept help: practice letting go of things you don't need to control. Delegate more. Ask for help when you need it. Make time for doing things that replenish you.

9

Using Yoga with Other Modalities for Fertility Support

Many complementary practices work well with a fertility yoga practice to help enhance fertility. Acupuncture and Traditional Chinese Medicine are used alone as well as in conjunction with yoga and ART (Assisted Reproductive Technology). In fact, some reproductive endocrinologists work with acupuncturists who will come into the office on the day of transfer while you are going through an IVF cycle.

Fertility abdominal massage is another technique that can be very useful either alone or in conjunction with the other methodologies mentioned. This technique involves manual stimulation of the reproductive organs through a massage of the abdominal area. The massage can help with a number of issues related to this area of the body, but has been very effective for women who are experiencing difficulty trying to conceive.

This chapter will explore each of these practices and how they may be used to help enhance your fertility. Hypnotherapy, talk therapy, and consulting with a life coach are also explained and explored in this chapter. At the end of the chapter, you will find suggestions for talking with family members about your fertility journey.

ACUPUNCTURE

Traditional Chinese Medicine is a system of health care that employs acupuncture, dietary advice, Chinese massage, and moxa (heat treatment) to help clear blockages in the body and enhance fertility and conception. Acupuncturists look at the body as a system, and emphasize balancing the Yin and Yang energies. They assess the interactions of various substances like Qi (pronounced chee), the word used for vital life energy, and blood, the denser lubricating fluid of the body. The Qi is considered to be the Yang force in the body, while the blood is the Yin component. When blockage occurs in the flow of Qi or blood, it can create an imbalance, resulting in disease or pain. Acupuncture treatments use tiny needles into the skin along meridians or energy centers to unblock the obstructions. This encourages the free flow of Qi and blood which leads to optimal health.

One Acupuncturist's Thoughts on Fertility Issues

According to acupuncturist Ruijuan Liu, the reason we are seeing such an increase in infertility is due to the age at which women are trying to conceive as well as toxicity in the body. Kidney/ Yin and Yang energy dominate reproduction and start to decline after age 35. Acupuncture and Chinese herbs rejuvenate the kidney energy, helping to enhance the function of the reproductive system. Toxicity in the body can be caused by diet and lifestyle choices as well as environmental factors. The chemicals we are exposed to from the air we breathe, medication, and cleaning products are a few factors which can cause toxicity. Acupuncture can help reduce the levels of toxicity in the body. Every patient is different and is born with a certain weakness or imbalance in the body. However, there are lifestyle choices which can cause an increase in these imbalances. Our 21st century, fast-paced lifestyle of multitasking and "doing" can cause stagnation in the liver. Cold drinks and overwork/exertion can cause a spleen deficiency. Chinese herbs and acupuncture help to bring the Qi back to these energy centers so that the energy can flow more freely and conception can take place. According to Dr. Liu, if you don't have good soil, the seed cannot grow.

For thousands of years, Chinese medicine has had a strong focus on women's health and fertility. One reason for this is that having children has always been highly valued in Chinese culture. Many fertility clinics now encourage their patients to seek out acupuncture as a supportive component of their care. Acupuncture can also help specifically with conditions like high FSH, thin uterine lining, ovulatory problems, low sperm counts, painful menstrual cycles, and stress or anxiety. For example, Chinese medicine seeks to improve the quality of the eggs, which can become weak due to depletion of the kidney, spleen and liver systems. Modern lifestyles, stress and poor diet can all stress these systems. Once these are rebalanced, the egg quality improves. Receiving acupuncture during an IVF cycle can help reduce the side effects from the fertility drugs, as well as create a more optimal environment for implantation. The stimulation from acupuncture can also boost the number of follicles produced when patients do acupuncture during an ART cycle. Like fertility yoga, acupuncture can help regulate hormone levels, reduce stress and help increase general well being.

When you see an acupuncturist he/she will review your history and ask many questions about how your body works. You may be asked questions such as when are you thirsty and if you get up in the night to urinate, or about the regularity of your menstrual cycles. These questions are designed to help make a diagnosis from a Chinese medical perspective, and you may hear phrases like Liver Qi stagnation, blood deficiency, or Kidney Yin deficiency, which can all be common when fertility is compromised.

In Traditional Chinese Medicine, treatment plans are very individualized, because two different people with the same symptoms may have different underlying problems. Your acupuncturist will come up with an individualized plan of action that may include dietary changes, herbs, and acupuncture treatments to support your goals. Acupuncture and fertility yoga together are very complementary, and are beneficial to both your physical and emotional well being.

A Few Basic Fertility-Supporting Practices from Chinese Medicine

Some basic fertility-supporting recommendations from Traditional Chinese Medicine, that are simple to implement, include:

- Choose warm food over cold food.
- Avoid drinking very cold liquids, and don't use ice in your drinks. Room temperature liquids, or hot liquids are recommended.
- Keep your feet warm, so always wear socks or slippers. A warm foot-bath before bed is recommended.

To find a qualified acupuncturist, you can ask your yoga instructor, doctor, or a friend who has gone through a similar situation. All acupuncturists should be state licensed and have passed the national exam through the National Certification Commission for Acupuncture and Oriental Medicine. A directory of certified acupuncturists can be found on the NCCAOM website. See the Resource Pages at the back of the book for more information.

FERTILITY ABDOMINAL MASSAGE

Fertility abdominal massage is another ancient healing method that was used for thousands of years by midwives, shaman, and other healers in many places around the world. The most popular form of this external massage was brought to the United States by Dr. Rosita Arvigo. Dr. Arvigo was trained by one of the last traditional Mayan shaman, Don Elijio Panti. She spent 10 years studying with him and combined what she learned from him with her naprapathic and herbal training to form the Arvigo Techniques of Maya Abdominal Therapy™. To find a therapist trained in the Arvigo Techniques of Maya Abdominal Therapy™, you can visit their website at www.arvigotherapy.com.[1]

This non-invasive, external massage helps put the reproductive organs, most specifically the uterus, back in its proper position in the body. The massage helps improve organ function by releasing physical and emotional congestion and bringing health and vitality back to the pelvic region. Before doing the massage, the therapist will ask many questions about your body and previous traumas or injuries that may have caused the uterus to shift from its optimal position. The therapists are looking to clear both physical and emotional congestion in the abdominal area. They may also make other recommendations about nutrition or other complementary practices to aid in their work. You can expect to spend up to two hours with the therapist on your first visit, with subsequent visits lasting about an hour. Many women feel that fertility abdominal massage, either by itself or in combination with yoga or ART, has played a very powerful role in helping them become pregnant.

HYPNOTHERAPY

Hypnotherapy involves dealing with emotional issues and obstacles at the level of the subconscious mind. The theory behind using hypnotherapy for fertility issues is that often, especially in cases of "unexplained infertility," no physical reason has been found to explain why pregnancy is not being achieved. However, the mind can have a strong influence on the health of the body, and emotional obstacles to pregnancy can be equally as important as physical problems. Hypnotherapy works to reduce the body's stress response by processing old subconscious issues that may be causing stress around trying to conceive. These old issues can be present as blocks even if our conscious mind appears very eager to attain pregnancy. The book *The Mind-Body Fertility Connection*, by James Schwarz explains more about using this modality, and offers suggestions for finding a therapist.[2]

COUNSELING AND LIFE COACHING

Counseling in the form of psychotherapy or talk therapy can be very helpful if you have been trying to conceive for a long time or have had a difficult time on your journey. Talking with another person who is not in the medical field and who can be objective about your situation may help you get more clear on your feelings, as well as help you make important decisions around your treatment options. Experiencing miscarriages or simply the normal highs and lows we go through each month when we are trying to conceive can impact emotional and mental well being. It is not uncommon to have strong feelings of sadness, anger, resentment and even jealousy, especially right after an unsuccessful treatment or a miscarriage. When talking with your spouse, friends or family members is not enough, it may be wise to look into finding a therapist or life coach who can help you work through your feelings of loss and sadness. There are many ways to find a therapist in your area. RESOLVE, the National Infertility Organization, has a list of mental health professionals and life coaches who deal specifically with fertility. You may also want to consult your insurance company, as therapy or counseling may be covered under your insurance plan. There are also many websites that can help you connect with a therapist or life coach. Please see the Resource Pages in the back of the book for a full list of websites and resources.

ASSISTED REPRODUCTIVE TECHNOLOGY (ART)

Assisted Reproductive Technology is an option offered by fertility clinics for couples who are having difficulty conceiving. The rule of thumb that the clinics typically recommend is that you seek the help of a doctor when you have not become pregnant within a year of trying to conceive naturally if you are under 35 years of age and within six months if you are over 35 years of age.[3]

When you visit a reproductive endocrinologist, they will do a series of tests to see what factors, both male and female, may be affecting your ability to conceive.

Each fertility practice has their own approach to treatment, and their pregnancy success rates are published each year on the CDC website. The following list provides some information on common treatment protocols. This list is by no means exhaustive. We offer it here to give you an idea of which treatments are commonly used in conjunction with yoga and the other techniques described in this chapter.

Clomid/IUI: Many practices will advise you to start taking a drug such as, clomiphene citrate (Clomid), or letrozole (Femara). These may be taken either with or without assistance in the form of an IUI (intrauterine insemination), as a fairly non-invasive form of treatment. Clomid is a synthetic drug that stimulates ovulation by blocking estrogen receptors in the hypothalamus. The hypothalamus responds by secreting GnRH and stimulates the pituitary gland to produce FSH (follicle stimulating hormone) and LH (lutenizing hormone). The IUI consists of injecting sperm, which has been carefully prepared in the lab, directly into the uterus through a catheter.

IUI with Injectable Drugs: Depending on your age, the outcome of your test results, and the practice you are working with, you may be advised to use injectable drugs to stimulate the ovaries, combined with an IUI (intrauterine insemination) as a form of treatment. The injectable drugs are the same stimulation drugs used with in vitro fertilization (IVF). A much lower dose of the drugs is needed since the goal is to produce only 2–3 eggs. Unless special circumstances exist, fertility clinics often recommend trying IUI's before moving on to IVF (in vitro fertilization).

IVF (in vitro fertilization): This is a more invasive treatment which requires stimulation of the ovaries, followed by a procedure to remove the oocytes (eggs) that have grown as a result of the stimulation. Sperm from the husband/partner or a donor are carefully prepared by an embryologist and placed in a petri dish with the eggs. Sometimes a procedure called ICSI (intra cytoplasmic sperm injection) is used, which involves injecting a single sperm into the egg to get better fertilization rates. Once the eggs are fertilized, the embryos begin to divide and are placed back into the uterus via a catheter between 2 and 5 days after the egg retrieval. The number of embryos transferred depends on a number of factors, including the quality of the embryos, as higher quality embryos have greater fertilization rates. The more embryos that are transferred, the more likely that pregnancy will occur. However, transferring several embryos also increases the chance of a multiple gestation and a high risk pregnancy. If there are embryos left over, clinics will offer cryopreservation (freezing) so that the embryos can be used for subsequent IVF cycles.[4]

Collaborative Reproduction/Donor Egg: This treatment option is often recommended by fertility clinics if the typical IVF protocol does not work, or if the doctor believes that the woman's eggs are not viable for a healthy pregnancy. Egg donation is one of several techniques that require a third party in order to have a baby. Others include sperm donation, embryo adoption, traditional adoption, and using a gestational carrier or surrogate. While IVF with a donor egg has very good success rates, it is also quite costly and presents ethical, emotional and psychological considerations.[5] To learn more about this and other forms of ART, see the Resource Pages in the back of the book for a list of helpful books and websites.

Jill's Story

Doing fertility treatments can be very exciting but also scary. We often don't realize what we are getting into when we go down this path, and I hope for your sake you don't have to go too far down this road to become pregnant. One of the reasons I began teaching fertility yoga was to help other women deal with the stress of fertility treatments and trying to conceive in general. When I did my first Clomid/IUI, I just assumed that it would work. I can remember how devastated I was when I got my period that month. Each treatment got progressively more stressful as I continued down the road. I felt like so much was riding on the treatment and each negative pregnancy test was making me more and more depressed. I felt like something was wrong with Me. What did I do wrong that this wasn't working? I kept blaming myself for not going to the doctor sooner or for drinking too much coffee or alcohol. My husband and I were fighting a lot as he felt so helpless and just wanted me to get pregnant and feel better. The only solace I found was in my yoga and meditation practice and the support group that I was going to once a month. If you have not found support through yoga, friends or a support group, I highly recommend going to Resolve's website (www.resolve.org.) and finding a yoga class or support group in your area. You will find more information about doing yoga while going through fertility treatments as well as a stress relieving yoga practice in Chapter 6 of this book.

SUGGESTIONS FOR FRIENDS AND FAMILY

Talking about your fertility journey with friends and family can be both challenging and comforting. Well-meaning friends or family members may make a comment like, "If you just relax, you'll get pregnant," without realizing how this statement minimizes what you are going through. Conversely, a friend or family member may say just the right thing like, "I know you and Tom are going to be wonderful parents regardless of how long it takes or how that baby comes to you." This section will give you suggestions about how to talk about your fertility challenges, as well advice you can share with friends and family on how to better understand your situation.

Deciding on how much you want to share about your difficulties trying to conceive is a completely personal decision that

Kim's Story

I went to visit my OB/GYN after a year of trying to conceive and not getting pregnant. He did some tests and told me that he thought I might have a mild case of PCOS and referred me to a reproductive endocrinologist. While I was in the midst of the tests and trying to find out why I was not getting pregnant, a family member got married. At the wedding reception, the bride and groom told me and my husband that "the race was on" to see which couple might get pregnant first. I remember going to the bathroom and crying hysterically as I knew I was already losing this so-called race. These family members didn't know the extent of what my husband and I were going through, and were just trying to be funny, but that didn't help how devastated I felt at the time.

is best discussed between you and your partner. You may have different feelings about who you feel comfortable talking to about your situation and how much you want to share. If you decide to talk openly about your situation, you may find the following tips from Resolve, the National Infertility Association, helpful.

1. Decide how much detail you and your partner want to share. Respect each other's need for privacy about certain details.

2. It may help to rehearse exactly what you are going to say. Decide on specific words or phrases to use, such as "infertility" or "we are trying to get pregnant and seem to be having a problem."

3. Pick a time to talk when people are not rushed or distracted. Make sure it is a private place where you won't feel embarrassed to show emotion.

4. Explain that infertility is a life crisis, and that 1 in 8 couples, or more than 7 million people experience it.

5. Let them know how they can support you—whether you want phone calls, questions, etc.

6. Explain that you may need a break from family gatherings, and that it isn't about them—it's about using your energy wisely.

7. Tell them that you will share results about a treatment or procedure when you feel up to it, and not to ask about pregnancy tests or treatment results.[6]

One of the best ways that friends and family members can support you is by educating themselves about infertility. Most people don't know a lot about the subject other than what they may have seen on TV or have heard from other people. And people assume that if they got pregnant without any trouble, then so can you. In my experience, it's not that those people are all insensitive jerks; they just don't know the facts about infertility. If you are comfortable, you can help educate family members yourself, or direct them to helpful websites or books found in the Resources Pages at the back of this book.

Another way that friends and family can support you is by listening. People often feel that they have to say the right thing, which is hard to do when it comes to this topic. Often what we need is a compassionate friend who will just listen to what we are going through without offering advice. I have found that it's best if you are very clear with your friends and family about not really needing advice, but rather just someone to listen to your experience.

Sometimes, you just need to spend time with friends and family without talking about or being reminded of what you are going through. Again, find the friends and family members that you feel you can communicate with most honestly and openly, and try to spend time with them, letting them know that you are not up for discussing your situation.

The following list is something you may want to print out and share with your close friends and family. It's a list of the common statements and advice made by people with the best intentions, unaware that saying these things may cause more harm than good. You can let them know that it's okay if they've said any of these things to you and your partner in the past. You might tell them you are just making a simple request, and letting them know about some things they can avoid saying to anyone they know who might be having difficulty conceiving.

Things That Are Not Helpful to Hear

1. Just relax, and you will get pregnant.
2. Stop thinking about it and you will get pregnant.
3. Go on vacation, and you will you get pregnant.
4. Why don't you just adopt?
5. Maybe you guys just aren't meant to be parents.
6. I'm sure it will happen when you least expect it.
7. I know someone who adopted and then got pregnant.
8. Why don't you try IVF?
9. Why don't you try egg donor or a surrogate?
10. There are worse things that can happen.

While this is not a comprehensive list of all the wrong things to say (people can always come up with more variations!) these are some of the more common and difficult things to hear, even if the person saying them has the best of intentions.

Now, here is a list of some of the right things to say to someone who is having difficulty trying to get pregnant. Again, this list is not comprehensive, but is just meant to help people who really don't know what to say.

Helpful Things to Say

1. I'm sorry that you are going through this. It must be really hard.
2. I'm here for you no matter what happens.
3. If you need someone to talk to, I will listen and not offer advice unless you ask me for it.
4. I love you.
5. I wish you didn't have to go through this.
6. Is there anything I can do to help you through this difficult time?
7. I wish I had the right thing to say to help you feel better.
8. How can I best support you during this difficult time?
9. I understand if you can't make all of the family functions during this time. You and your partner have to do what's best for you right now.
10. If there is something I say or have said that was painful for you to hear, please let me know so I can avoid saying it again.

Again, these are just some suggestions to help the people who are closest to you support you and your partner during a difficult time. If you want to individualize the list to meet your specific situation, by all means do. Personalizing your top 10 list of "right and wrong things to say" may be therapeutic for you and your partner, and may be really appreciated by the people closest to you.

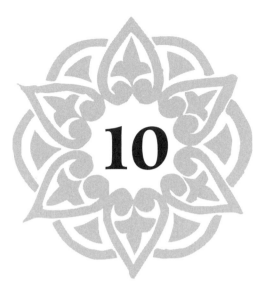

10

Success Stories

In this chapter, you will learn that there are many different ways to fulfill your dream of having a child. We are very grateful that several of our students have been willing to share their fertility stories to include in the final chapter of this book. There are many more stories like this. Together, we have had well over a thousand women take our Yoga for Fertility classes. We are continually humbled by the lessons we learn again and again from our students. Here are just a few:

■ How to believe in and follow our own intuition when many "experts" are telling us something different.
■ How to use courage and discipline to make changes in our lives, in order to support our goals and values.
■ How to persevere in the face of sometimes daunting odds.

■ How to focus on the positive by choosing to do so.
■ How to find the support we need when the path is challenging.

The following "success stories" all have happy endings, although these students ended up taking many different paths to arrive there. In reading these, you may recognize some of your own path. If so, we hope you may discover inspiration and ideas to help you along the way.

WENDY'S STORY

We had been married about two years when we decided it was time to start trying to have a child. At the time, I was 32, and had never had really normal monthly cycles. We tried to conceive for about a year, and then I consulted my regular doctor, who basically told me there was nothing wrong, and we should keep trying. When we still had no luck, I went to an OB/Gyn, who said essentially the same thing. I kept thinking that someone should be able to give me some answers, so I consulted several more doctors. I got suggestions to cut down on my running and exercise, and to start eating better, which I did. But no one really could tell me why we were having so much trouble. It reminded me of going to job interviews, but every time I thought they would give me the job, they said "No, sorry" but wouldn't tell me why! I got very frustrated and cried a lot during this time.

Eventually, my doctor told me I had PCOS (polycystic ovarian syndrome), and an OB/Gyn put me on clomid and Metformin. I didn't like being on so much medication, and besides, my intuition told me that this was not the answer for me. I was so confused, and really stopped trusting what the doctors said. I felt like everyone had given up on me. I started to feel very lost, and like I was really out on my own trying to figure out how to fix my problem. I hadn't really told any of my friends what I was going through, because it seemed like they were all getting pregnant, no problem. In fact, during this time I had several friends stop by to "surprise me" with their pregnancy announcements. While I wanted to feel joy for them, I couldn't help feeling sad and angry. I started isolating myself from many of my friends.

Finally, I confided in one friend, and discovered that she had also had difficulty getting pregnant. She encouraged me to join Lynn's Yoga for Fertility class. I was skeptical, as I had never done yoga before, but she said I could go with her. At first, I didn't think I was getting much benefit

from the class, but I kept going because my friend wanted me to. Then, after about three months of class and doing the yoga at home most days, I started to really feel different. I had more energy, my mood was more positive, and I just felt some kind of "warmth" in my body that hadn't been there before. Even though I had always done a lot of exercise, including running up to 25 miles a week, I felt myself getting stronger in a very different way. I also felt that the yoga practice validated my feeling that I needed to tune in to my own intuition about my body. I also decided to try some of the other options Lynn had mentioned in class, including acupuncture and fertility abdominal massage.

About this time, I decided to take a month off of "trying" and go on a trip to China with my mom. My mom was questioning me about the medications I was taking, and although I actually agreed with her, I still resented her questions. It was a good trip, but I found that I really missed my yoga practice, which was hard to do while traveling.

Almost immediately after we got back, I decided to stop taking the clomid and Metformin. I also decided to attend the Women's Fertility Retreat that Lynn and Carol were offering, which turned out to be really transformational for me, for many reasons. I learned the practice of "mindfulness" and cognitive restructuring, which helped me get out of my negative thought patterns. And I found such a supportive group of women there! It was such a relief to know that I could say whatever I needed to say about my situation, and those women would know exactly what I meant. I found myself letting go of my stress about my fertility issues, and I became able to enjoy life again.

Shortly after returning home from the retreat, I started feeling tired and a little nauseous, but I didn't pay too much attention, until my acupuncturist told me my pulses were like those of a pregnant lady. I went home and took a home pregnancy test, and when it was positive, I figured it must have been a faulty test. After the second one gave the same result, though, I scheduled a blood test with my doctor. When that also came back positive, I had to really believe it! I was pregnant at last, having conceived naturally, at age 34, after more than two years of trying.

In retrospect, I feel a big contributor to my success was keeping an open mind and being willing to try non-traditional approaches, such as yoga, acupuncture, massage, and the mind/body techniques we learned on the retreat. Also important was being open to my own journey, instead of doing things just because someone else had told me I should. I had to believe in the validity of my own intuition. My main recommendations to other women facing fertility challenges would be to stay patient, stay positive, and don't be ashamed of your situation. If I hadn't finally started sharing what was going on with a few friends, I would not have found out about the things that helped me so much, such as the yoga class and the retreat. I have been telling all my friends who are trying to get pregnant to go to the yoga for fertility class, and so far, *all* of them have gotten pregnant—even the ones who were skeptical about trying yoga!

P.S. After the positive pregnancy test, I joined Lynn's prenatal yoga class, and continued doing yoga at home during my pregnancy. I had a pretty quick (4 hours) and "easy" birth, which I attribute to the yoga and especially the breathing practices we did in class. My beautiful son had some colic for the first few months, but he is feeling better now, and things have gotten easier. I might even consider trying for baby #2 at some point in the future, now that I have seen that my intuition was right, and I am able to conceive naturally.

ANNA'S STORY

I met my husband in the summer of 2010, when I was 41. We started talking kids right away. We both knew we wanted kids and we knew we needed to get started soon. I had always had kind of irregular periods, so I decided to go to my OB/GYN and get some basic testing done. When the FSH test came back at 15, my OB was totally discouraging. She told me that probably my only chance to get pregnant was to use a donor egg. I was absolutely shocked. We hadn't even started trying yet, and all of a sudden I was told that I had absolutely no chance of getting pregnant on my own.

We decided to go to a fertility clinic. The doctor there was slightly more positive—until my FSH testing came back at 24. Then he said they would not consider doing IVF, and that my chances to conceive using IUI's were about 5%.

We were devastated and I felt very depressed and anxious. I saw a flyer for a Mind/Body Program at the fertility clinic, and thought this might help me, so I signed up for the 10-week program. Lynn taught Yoga for Fertility at one of the sessions, and I signed up for her weekly classes. I found it so helpful to be with other women who could understand how I felt, and the yoga and meditation helped me feel better. It was like getting my batteries recharged every week, and also got me back on an even keel so that I could begin doing my own research on what other avenues might be out there to help me.

In the spring of 2011, I added a nutritionist to my "fertility team", and based on her advice, I stopped drinking coffee, reduced my sugar and dairy intake, and upped my veggie intake. I was already buying organic food whenever possible, but my diet improved a lot with her help. I even started juicing, and going to the local organic restaurant for wheat grass juices— basically I did anything that anyone had mentioned might help with fertility! We were also busy planning our wedding for later that spring.

We decided to go back to the fertility clinic and try one round of IUI with injectable hormones, but the IUI was cancelled mid-cycle, when the doctor felt the follicles were developing too slowly. We decided we should go ahead and try naturally, anyway, but I was so discouraged. The IUI was the only option the clinic had offered us, and now it appeared that my ovaries weren't even in good enough shape for this option to work.

I called Lynn to do a private consultation. I really felt I was running out of options. As I sat in her yoga room relating how the IUI hadn't worked, I couldn't help crying. I felt like our dreams of having a family were already shattered, before we were even married. Lynn asked me some questions, like what day of my cycle I was on now, and whether we had tried naturally after the cycle was cancelled. Then she said "I'd like you to go home and take a pregnancy test, before I give you any yoga practice to do. Call me afterwards." I was surprised, but figured she was just being extra cautious.

Twenty minutes later, I called her back. "You're not going to believe this! I'm pregnant!" I had also been trying to text my husband at work, but couldn't reach him with this unbelievable news. Later that day, I learned that he had come home after I had left, and had seen the test stick with the positive lines on it. He said his thought was "Wow, wouldn't it be nice if that were true." But of course with all of our recent bad news, he didn't for a moment believe that it might be true.

When I met with Lynn again, she told me that as she sat talking with me that morning, she had an overwhelming urge to say to me, "Anna, why are you crying? Everything is going to be fine. You will be pregnant at your wedding!" She sent me home because she had such a strong intuition that I was already pregnant. She later told me she had never before sent someone home to take a pregnancy test. And it was true—I was pregnant at our wedding two months later, and have since joined Lynn's prenatal yoga class. I'm at 36 weeks as I write this!

I feel that my choice to focus on the positive, rather than the negative, helped me be successful in the face of the Western medical community's discouraging prognosis. When the doctor told me I had a 5% chance of getting pregnant, I figured OK, well there is at least a 5% chance that I will get pregnant—why shouldn't I be the one that falls into that 5%? I was also encouraged by a section I found in Toni Weschler's book *Taking Charge of Your Fertility*. This section wasn't even in the "fertility" part of the book, but in the "preventing conception" part—where it said that you needed to take precautions unless and until you were actually in menopause, because you were definitely fertile until then.

I also took hope from a statement Lynn made in class one time: that everyone in her classes eventually finds a solution that is right for them. While many women get pregnant, some do that by using donor eggs, or adopting embryos, and others decide to adopt a child. Some choose to stop pursuing pregnancy, and to incorporate their desire to parent in other ways in their life. Although I was offered lots of negative opinions, I decided to focus on the things that were telling me that it WAS possible for me to get pregnant.

GEORGIA'S STORY

After one miscarriage and then almost a year of trying to conceive without any success, we sought the help of a fertility clinic. I had all of the routine tests and everything came back normal; nothing could point to any signs of a potential issue. We had unexplained infertility. To help speed things along, I began Clomid to help increase egg production. My body responded well at first to the medication and then the side effects began to take their toll and it was determined Clomid was not the best medication for me. After several months off the medication in an attempt to get my body back to "normal," we conceived naturally for the second time. Unfortunately, this pregnancy also ended in an early miscarriage. I underwent a D&C so further testing could be done to try and help identify potential answers. All tests showed the fetus was healthy. The only answer given was we were having bad luck and there was no reason why we shouldn't be able to get pregnant and carry a healthy baby to term.

Wanting to do anything in our power to help with a successful pregnancy, we enlisted the help of several specialists— some for how to cope with our situation on an emotional level and others from a medical perspective beyond the traditional Western approach. We enrolled in a couple's Mind Body Wellness Class that provided a safe environment for openly talking about infertility and our specific journey. The class introduced us to several tools and techniques to help with mitigating stress and feelings of anxiety and offered ideas on how to more effectively increase communication between ourselves and friends and family. It was in the Mind Body class where I was introduced to Yoga for Fertility.

Stress and depression continued to be the biggest challenges for me. To help cope, I started seeing an abdominal massage therapist. I've never been one to do things for myself and at first thought that going to massage seemed excessive—I was wrong. I had an amazing experience with abdominal massage and didn't realize what a specialty area this was and how so many things in the body are intrinsically linked. The massage helped with the stress reduction and I strongly feel prepared my body to help support a healthy pregnancy. In addition to massage, I began taking the Yoga for Fertility class.

The yoga class offered me a place where I could go each week and be among a group of women who understood what I was going through. It was a safe environment for sharing and learning. The yoga was just the right pace for me (a beginner) and provided me the needed breathing and relaxation techniques. It was a class that I looked forward to every week because I knew I could decompress and forget about everything else (even if was only for an hour and 15 minutes). I also was introduced to an amazing group of women who I remain close with to this day; over a year after my child was born.

Six months after the second miscarriage, we conceived again without the aid of any medications. Early ultrasounds showed that this pregnancy was not viable due to a very low heartbeat and ended in miscarriage number three. By this point we were devastated and left looking for answers. Another D&C was done and this pregnancy was identified as having a chromosome abnormality. We both had a full blood panel workup to determine if we were carriers of anything genetic or otherwise that may be preventing a successful pregnancy.

The only thing identified was that I was heterozygous for MTHFR (an enzyme involved in folic acid metabolism in the body). Mutations in the MTHFR gene can affect how a person's body processes homocysteine, an amino acid found in the blood. MTHFR has been identified as a possible contributing factor to recurrent miscarriage. Our particular fertility clinic did not recognize MTHFR as a possible reason for the recurrent miscarriage. *(Author's note: see Chapter 8 for more information on MTHFR).*

At this point, we also started working with a naturopath who specialized in fertility who was able to more thoroughly explain MTHFR and its ties to miscarriage. We received a different medical perspective and were offered reassurance that we were taking the right steps for getting as healthy as we could to help with conception. We also received recommendations for a healthier eating plan which was complemented by various vitamins, and which made us both feel much better. I was prescribed special folic acid to help support my fourth pregnancy, which ended up being a success. We had decided to keep trying naturally, and one month following the third miscarriage, we conceived again. This one ended in the birth of a healthy, vibrant baby daughter.

Concurrent to working with the naturopath, I was also seeing an acupuncturist who specializes in pregnancy and fertility. After one session, I could tell a difference in my anxiety and stress level and felt that I was doing something good for both my baby and myself. I continued to use acupuncture throughout my pregnancy.

While the journey was difficult and tested us on so many levels, both individually and as a couple, we had a very positive experience working with the fertility clinic. I have no complaints or regrets. It was frustrating not getting the answers we were looking for; however, the experience and how we were treated by the clinic was all very positive.

Participating in activities such as Yoga for Fertility, acupuncture and massage helped me feel like I had some control over the situation. So often when you are having fertility challenges things are out of your control, and these activities allowed me to be the one in charge. I felt empowered that I was choosing to do something good for my mind and my body.

One thing I learned during our journey is that it is possible to have a family if you want one, it just might not be the way you had originally imagined. I kept what we were going through hidden for a long time and was embarrassed to talk about it, thinking there was something wrong with me. Know that you are not alone; there are so many people struggling in a similar way who understand what you are going through. Finding a group to talk about what I was experiencing was extremely helpful and kept me motivated as I heard about their success stories. I feel blessed that I now have my own success story to share.

We have one amazing daughter and recently found out that we are expecting baby number two. Miracles do happen.

SUZETTE'S STORY

I met my husband on a climbing trip, when I was 39 and he was 37. We both knew we wanted kids, and so we started trying right away once we knew we intended to be together long term. I actually got pregnant easily, but then had a very early miscarriage. After trying a few more months, we decided to at least get checked out by my regular OB/Gyn. She thought all looked good, and had us try a few cycles using clomid. After this didn't work, she referred us to a fertility clinic for further consultation. At this point, I had just turned 41, but my FSH levels and all my testing looked fine. I had been doing a lot of climbing and Pilates, and I felt in great shape.

The reproductive endocrinologist suggested that we go straight to IVF. Because of my age, she felt that we should move quickly to give ourselves the best chance of success. When the first IVF round didn't work, she talked to us about the possibility of using donor eggs for a second cycle. We weren't prepared to try that yet, and decided to take a few months break, and then try another IVF cycle.

At this point, I noticed some flyers for a Mind/Body program at the clinic. When I called about it, the program had already started, but the director referred me to Lynn's yoga for fertility classes. I had read a lot about how stress could have a negative impact on fertility, and how yoga could help reduce your body's reaction to stress. I started doing individual yoga sessions with Lynn, and practicing the routines she gave me every morning. Lynn also referred me to an acupuncturist who was very experienced working with women undergoing IVF. She gave me weekly treatments, and also gave me some supplements that help to support the reproductive

system, and a heart-shaped stone to help me keep my focus on my fertility goals. At the same time, I started working with an energy healer. All of these women shared a lot of knowledge with me about the IVF process, and how to best support my fertility going into it.

When we started the second IVF round, I felt I had a "support team" behind me, and also that I had been able to take some control of a process that otherwise had felt very out of my control. I had not liked the feeling of just handing my body over to the fertility doctors, even if they were very skilled. It seemed like they were just overriding all of the wisdom that I knew my body possessed about how to make babies. But now I felt I was able to be a bigger part of the process.

Although the quantity was about the same, the embryos were better quality than what I had produced in the first IVF round. This time, I had acupuncture both just before and just after my embryo transfer, which had been shown in one German study to have improved the IVF success rates. And I used some of the visualizations Lynn had given me.

As I was lying there after my post-transfer acupuncture treatment, I suddenly felt a strong bolt of energy that came in through the top of my head and kind of rolled down my body. It was followed by another bolt that was more gentle, and which I can only describe as moving back and forth the way a fish swims. In hindsight, I believe this reflected the energy of my twins coming into my body—my daughter is very direct and forceful, and my son has an easier going, more organic approach to life. And when they were born, she came out first, and he followed.

As you can already see, this story had a very happy ending. I continued with my hour of yoga practice every morning throughout my pregnancy. Lynn modified the routine as I got bigger, but I was able to still do many poses up until the day before my babies were born. Although C-sections tend to be very common with twins, I was able to have a scheduled vaginal delivery in week 37. The doctors and nurses were so impressed with how the birth had gone that several of them asked me what I had done to prepare, and I said "Lots of yoga!"

I feel strongly that both the yoga and the acupuncture contributed to my successful pregnancy and birth. I would encourage other women to start both of these early—as soon as you are thinking of trying to conceive—as the benefits are really cumulative. In addition, I made some dietary changes, such as giving up caffeine (hard!), and adding more dark green leafy vegetables to my diet. I had already been eating organic foods for some time, so I just tried to eat as much healthy food as I could. Also, I was fortunate that, in my job as a university professor, I had some control over my work schedule during the quarter when I was doing my 2nd IVF procedure and was able to reduce my teaching load during the final trimester of my pregnancy. I would encourage other women to make any stress-reducing lifestyle changes they can, at least during the time when they are trying to conceive.

PRITI'S STORY

For 5 years, I worked with a fertility clinic. I had several cycles of IUI with medication and 4 IVF cycles done. I would say that I had at least 10 IUI cycles. I never wanted a month to go by without trying something. I also tried 1 IVF cycle in India. I thought that going to India might be the magic,

but it didn't work. I believed in God and the doctors and never worried or was very bothered by all of this. I just kept trying.

Throughout my journey, I was doing yoga. For the last year, I started acupuncture. I also got a massage called Clear Passage Therapy™. The Clear Passage treatments that I did were over 2 hours away and my husband and I drove down there at least 10 times so I could have these treatments. They were pretty costly too; $5000 for 20 treatments and I did them all. I stopped caffeine, took a very simple job near my home. Other than that I kept myself positive and upbeat for which yoga helped a lot. I feel that yoga and acupuncture were the most beneficial of all of the complementary approaches that I tried. I am continuing both yoga and acupuncture for overall wellbeing now.

In the Fertility Yoga classes, I met other women on the same journey which gave me a sense of community. Not everyone in my class was going through fertility treatments, but we were all working towards the end result of having a baby. The poses designed for this purpose kept me calm and hopeful that I am doing something towards the goal.

In the end, though I did not have a biological child and adopted my beautiful daughter Isha from India, I had a sense of peace when I made the decision to adopt. I firmly believe that my yoga practice helped me in this. For that I am grateful for yoga and my teacher Jill. When I went to India to bring my daughter home, I practiced yoga there. Yoga, acupuncture and meditation/prayer contributed to my success in achieving my dream of becoming a parent, by bringing home my daughter.

The advice I would give to women who are having difficulty trying to conceive is just accept the fact that doctors are not God. They will do their best. We have to do our part and remain calm and optimistic throughout our journey. Read a lot of self help books, pray and leave the rest to God.

VICKY'S STORY

My journey is one awe-inspiring journey, so I've been told. At age 39 I began to feel desperate about having a baby. It was not happening on its own, so I went to a fertility doctor. They performed some tests and after an HSG they said we may get pregnant on our own. It actually happened!!! But the excitement was short-lived; I ended up having a miscarriage just before turning 40.

After that the docs threw in the towel. No less than four doctors from various clinics told me that my journey to motherhood would not be with my own eggs. But my husband kept insisting that since I had a miscarriage I could get pregnant and that we should try with my own eggs. Nevertheless, all clinics turned me away when I said I wanted to try IVF with my eggs. We even went all the way to a top clinic specializing in "advanced maternal age" in Colorado. But they also refused to do IVF with my eggs. Returning home was a low point in my journey. However, I had heard that a big reason clinics don't want to do IVF with older women is that they don't want to affect their success rates. They were just going by their statistics; it didn't really have much to do with whether or not **I** could get pregnant. That thought encouraged me.

I did finally find a clinic that would give it a try with my eggs, and that was really only because I found out that the head nurse was a friend of mine from college. But before that I spent months preparing my body for IVF.

First I did Qi Gong, which was really helpful with centering. Then, my husband and I joined Lynn's Yoga for Fertility class. Both of these practices are transforming. The yoga practice was a part of the journey that was the fun part. Yoga felt relaxing and calming, and it became part of my daily ritual. If I missed a day I felt it. It was helpful socially as well. We met other couples in class who were on the same journey, which made the road less lonely. We learned tips from each other and developed camaraderie.

I also started acupuncture, when I heard about that through yoga class. The first acupuncturist I went to was a bad fit. I then found someone who really cared and knew what she was doing, since fertility was a big part of her practice. She put me on a special diet, which omitted certain foods. She told me to eat organic non-packaged foods, and of course boiling up Chinese herbs became part of my daily routine. I read many books, including *The Infertility Cure,* by Randine Lewis and *Inconceivable,* which were very helpful and informative.

I tried as much as possible to eliminate all stress from my life. This was difficult to do when faced with fertility issues, but Qi Gong and yoga helped in dealing with the stress. Also, I was not working, so that helped. My acupuncturist had me omit caffeine, sugar and alcohol from my diet. I took many vitamins, including grape seed extract and fish oil. Exercise was to be non-vigorous, per my acupuncturist.

When I had the green light from my acupuncturist, we started our IVF protocol. We had to travel by airplane to the clinic, which was in another state, so we rented a condo and stayed about three weeks (our vacation). I made sure to come early enough and leave as late as possible so as to keep myself calm and not do anything that might disrupt the little embryos.

After all my preparation, I got pregnant on the first round of IVF using my own eggs (by now I was 41). At age 42, I gave birth to a healthy baby boy. As I had been told by multiple doctors that this wasn't going to be possible, I consider this baby as my über-miracle! A few years later I got pregnant naturally with my second child, at age 43. I gave birth at age 44 to a healthy baby girl. This baby is my traditional miracle!

I feel that one of the biggest contributors to my success was that I made a decision to give it my all. I took on the challenge and I sacrificed a lot to get to that place where my body's fertility clock was turned back. I poured my body, mind and spirit into becoming fertile. I became a disciplined fertility warrior. Yet, I had to let go of control, allow my acupuncturist to work her magic (skill), and allow the yoga and Qi gong to subtly work on my body. I tried to stay calm, eat right and **believe**.

My recommendations for others trying to get pregnant include staying positive, and finding support. I had a mantra and I constantly had to remind myself to think positive. I also made a fertility "altar" next to my bed, so that I would see positive reminders every morning and every night. I wore a necklace that said "Miracles happen every day," to remind myself that I could also have a "miracle" occur.

A friend who had gone through IVF before me gave me a piece of advice. She said, "You need a cheerleader. I'll be your cheerleader." My husband and this friend were my cheerleaders. Most of us going through this journey keep it very private and thus we can feel isolated and alone. Do find a good friend or family member who will be your cheerleader. And above all

your partner must be an active supportive participant. You need that support. By the way, I recommend getting your partner to practice yoga with you. For men it is helpful for fertility, too.

I know the success rate for a successful IVF after age 40 is very low according to the stats. But remember: doctors accept very few older women, so the data is minimal. If you turn back the clock by altering your body and lifestyle, and focus on the positive, you will greatly enhance your chances for success.

KATHY'S STORY

I met my husband when I was 38, and we both knew we wanted to start a family right away. So, even as we were preparing for our wedding, I went to see my OB/Gyn. My plan was to just have a routine check-up, and make sure all systems were "go." The doctor tested my FSH levels, and told me I had an FSH of 39, and since it would be difficult for me to get pregnant I should go to a fertility clinic. This is not what I expected to hear! I felt young, and looked young for my age, and I certainly had not thought I would have any trouble getting pregnant.

It turned out that at that time, my FSH was fluctuating from a low of 14 to a high of 39. At first, the fertility clinic talked to me about using a donor egg. This really shocked me as I was not even aware I had fertility issues—I was still on the pill! I wasn't willing to consider this option right off the bat, so the doctor at the fertility clinic decided to give my system a boost to see if I could get pregnant on my own before taking further procedural steps. She gave me supplemental estrogen as well as taking me off of birth control. At the same time, I began participating in a number of complementary medicine practices that I had heard could boost fertility, including shiatsu massage, yoga and dietary changes. I got pregnant within a month of starting the estrogen supplement. At the time I attributed it to my body work and mental focus. In retrospect, I'm guessing it had more to do with the hormone supplement and going off the pill. I had a normal pregnancy, and my daughter Lisa was born just as I turned 41. When she was about 9 months old, we decided not to waste time, and to start trying for number two.

Number two turned out to be a bit more difficult than number one. We did not return to the fertility clinic right away because I knew they would still be stuck on my high FSH level. Instead, I dove deeply into every kind of complementary medical practice I ran across that could help with my fertility. Over a period of several years, I worked with a Doctor of Oriental Medicine, doing herbs and acupuncture. I consulted a naturopathic physician who specialized in fertility. I had Maya abdominal massage, and Shiatsu massage. And I started taking Lynn's Yoga for Fertility classes.

It felt very good to have a "support team" like this working with me—a team who believed that I could be successful, and who had a vested interest in helping me get there. I was very thankful for their support, and also the support group I found at the yoga for fertility class. It was so helpful to have a group of women who understood what I was going through. And still, despite all of these efforts, it wasn't happening. I just wasn't getting pregnant. I started heading down the "failure" path and began to feel depressed. I was really down for a while because I had really felt like I could beat the odds again with a second pregnancy.

As a last ditch effort we attended a RESOLVE conference to see what our other options were and frankly, to decide if we would follow any path other than natural pregnancy or no pregnancy. We also went to a RESOLVE meeting where the donor egg coordinator from my fertility clinic was speaking. Instead of being turned off by the idea, as I thought I would be, listening to the coordinator and other people struggling as we were helped me to face my situation head on. Within a few days of the meeting, I had turned my thinking around and decided to let go of the self-pity and look at my situation from where I was rather than where I wished I was. I spoke to my acupuncture doctor about egg donation and instead of encouraging me to continue on the natural pregnancy path, she asked me how old I was. When I told her I was 44, she said, "Oh, well, in that case, do the donor egg." That was the final straw.

My husband and I started to think very hard about what we really wanted, and we realized that what we wanted most was a sibling for Lisa. The genetic connection was much less important to us than that goal. I have two adopted brothers, who are just as much my siblings as my biological sister. Knowing this was helpful in allowing me to grieve the loss of my dream to get pregnant with my own egg. Then, I was able to take the next step on a realistic path to the family I wanted.

We returned to the clinic and talked to the donor egg coordinator, who couldn't have been more wonderful. A little more FSH testing (hey, old habits die hard) and we were set on the donor egg option. Once we started down this route, it was a pretty smooth path. My daughter Dana was born about a year later. Now, there is no question that she is as much my daughter as Lisa, and the two are great friends—most of the time!

One of the things I learned from this long journey was how important it was to get past my expectations, so that I could really be open to looking at all my options. I had to allow my intuition to lead my steps, even as I did my research and gathered information. As a woman with a professional career, I was used to being a "doer," an achiever, someone that makes things happen. I think I fell into the trap of thinking "If I just do one more thing, I'll be successful." I realized that it was kind of an addictive process. I had to finally come to the point where I let go of the idea of *achieving*, and instead became okay with *receiving* the help I needed. In my case, the help was in the form of a donor egg. Like the other people I know who have built or added to their families through donor egg programs or adoption, I only wish I had done it sooner!

NANCY'S STORY

Ever since I can remember I wanted to have a child. It seemed to be a part of the fabric of my soul. After medical school, I chose Pediatric Anesthesiology as my specialty because working with children was the obvious path. By the time I met the man who would become my husband I was 38 years old but supremely confident that getting pregnant wouldn't be a problem. He had had a vasectomy but I was sure that modern medical science could handle that obstacle. We decided to try IVF as the easiest way to get pregnant and I began to prepare by joining Lynn's Yoga for Fertility class, and doing acupuncture. Our IVF failed and we were stunned. The IVF

process had been difficult and my intuitive sense was that this wasn't the way for us to have a baby.

So my husband had his vasectomy reversed with good results and once again, I was supremely confident that we would quickly be pregnant. Months went by and nothing happened. I began to reexamine my life. My job was full of stress and long hours. I was frequently on call and up all night taking care of very sick newborn babies. My energy was being completely drained taking care of other people's children in life and death situations. While I loved my job, I could see that it was preventing me from having a child of my own.

In a moment of crisis I went to my boss and told him that I was having a difficult time. He was immensely supportive and we found a way to change my schedule to decrease my exposure to small babies and cut back my hours. I stopped being on call overnight to eliminate the constant sleep deprivation, and found a wonderful psychotherapist who helped support me with the grief I was feeling. I continued my yoga practice and thought finally, I must be getting close to being pregnant.

Two years passed and nothing happened. I was diagnosed with a genetic mutation (MTHFR) and started on replacement methylfolate thinking this must be the problem. But still no pregnancy. The frustration and grief grew and I stopped going to yoga because the class became too difficult as so many people became pregnant. Everyone had a friend who had a miracle pregnancy. Where was my miracle? I had made dramatic life changes and still nothing. I began an exercise program and did an anti inflammatory diet which helped me lose 15 pounds. I quit drinking alcohol completely. Still nothing.

By now I was 43 years old and nothing had worked. The universe seemed to be playing a cruel joke on me and my mind began to entertain the thought that I might not ever have a child. Months went by and I started to envision my life without children. I stopped checking my ovulation and began planning for a different kind of future. My soul found a place of peace knowing that I had done everything possible to become pregnant and it just hadn't worked. I trusted that while the universe hadn't given me what I wanted, it had given me what I needed. My life was dramatically different than when I started my fertility journey in every way and I liked the person who I had become. I was healthier, happier and had found a type of contentment I didn't know was possible.

Then, my period was late. I was pregnant, at age 43, against all odds and with nothing changing other than me getting older! It seemed an impossible gift but gratitude became my daily mantra. I joined Lynn's prenatal yoga class, finally! The pregnancy progressed smoothly until we discovered the baby was small at 26 weeks and I was placed on bed rest for the remainder of the time. Once the shock was over, I found the blessings in my situation. Lots of sleep and time to read books. Incredible time with friends and family who came to keep me company. And the reminder again that life gives you what you need, not what you want.

P.S. I finished writing this just a few days before my beautiful son was born!

FINAL THOUGHTS FROM JILL AND LYNN

At one point in Nancy's story, she comments, "My life was dramatically different than when I started my fertility journey in every way and I liked the person who I had become. I was healthier, happier and had found a type of contentment I didn't know was possible." This sentiment has been echoed by so many of our students, and represents the silver lining to the cloud of fertility challenges. The lifestyle changes you choose to make as you prepare your body for pregnancy will very likely impact many areas of your life. The yoga and meditation practices you start as part of your fertility journey will also serve you well as a parent. Make the changes you are able to make. As we are reminded in one of the most ancient yoga texts, "No step on this path is ever wasted."[1]

We want to thank our students for sharing their stories which illustrate so beautifully that there are many different ways to fulfill your dream of having a child. This lesson from Georgia's story is one that we want to emphasize to those of you who have yet to realize your goal: "One thing I learned during our journey is that it is possible to have a family if you want one, it just might not be the way you had originally imagined."

Many of our students came to have their children in a much different way than they had thought or planned, which relates to the idea of "letting go" in yoga. When we say "letting go," we are not referring to letting go of the desire to fulfill your dreams. In fact, all of these women held strong to that desire and remained positive and steadfast despite many challenges and discouragements.

Wendy, in her story, points out another key lesson that she learned during her fertility challenges. She says, "Also important was being open to my own journey, instead of doing things just because someone else had told me I should. I had to believe in the validity of my own intuition." I myself had this experience over and over during the years I was trying to conceive, where I had to decide whether to believe "the experts" or to believe in my own intuition. I have since had a number of students tell me of having this struggle while dealing with fertility issues. In your process of trying to conceive, I would urge you to give at least equal weight to your own internal source of wisdom, as you do to information from outside "experts," no matter how learned they seem to be, or how many initials they have after their names. Your internal wisdom comes directly from Source, and as such, is extremely valuable, and rarely mistaken.

Deepak Chopra, M.D., author and co- founder of the Chopra Center for Well-being, reminds us that "What you focus on expands in your life," so it is vitally important to pay attention to what it is we are focusing on, and where we are putting our energy. We encourage you to stay focused and positive on your vision while "letting go" of the way that your dream gets realized. When we can let go in this way, the universe responds and gives us exactly what we need at just the right time.

Notes

CHAPTER 1

1. Tami Lynn Kent, *Wild Feminine* (Atria Books, 2011).
2. Alice Domar, *Conquering Infertility* (Viking Penguin, 2002), 28.
3. *Ibid.*, 25.
4. Science, November 12, 2010.

CHAPTER 2

1. Nalini Santanam, Presented at the annual meeting of the American Society for Reproductive Medicine, (2003).
2. Domar, *Conquering Infertility*, p. 29

CHAPTER 3

1. www.whattoexpect.com- "Ovulation: Five Ways to Tell You're Ovulating"

CHAPTER 7

1. Green and Green, 1977.
2. *Science Daily*, March 19, 2010.
3. Christine Northrup, *Women's Bodies, Women's Wisdom* (Bantam Books, 1994).
4. James Schwarz, *The Mind-Body Fertility Connection* (Llewellyn Publications, 2008) 165.
5. Marianne Szegedy-Maszak, "Mysteries of the Mind: Your unconscious is making your everyday decisions," *U.S. News and World Report*, February 28, 2005.

CHAPTER 8

1. Chavarro, J.E., et al, Human Reproduction, Feb. 28 2007, Vol. 22, Issue 5, p. 1340–1347.
2. *Ibid.*

3. *Ibid.*
4. www.shadygrovefertility.com/newsletter/effect-weight-fertility.
5. *ASRM Bulletin* 14 (18), March 16, 2012.
6. *Obstet Gynecology* 108 (2006): 938–46.
7. Berga S. L., et al. *Fertility & Sterility* 80 (2003): 891–976.
8. *Obstet Gynecology* 108 (2006): 938–46.
9. Alice Domar, *Conquering Infertility* (Viking Press, 2002) 272.
10. Chavarro, Willett, and Skerrit. From The Nurses' Study, *The Fertility Diet*.
11. Christine Northrup, *Women's Bodies, Women's Wisdom* (Bantam Books, 1994) 422.
12. Jeanie Lee Bussell, *Fully Fertile* (Findhorn Press, 2008) 75.

CHAPTER 9

1. www.arvigotherpy.com—The Arvigo Techniques of Maya Abdominal Massage Therapy.

2. James Schwarz, *The Mind-Body Fertility Connection*.
3. http://www.cdc.gov/art/—Centers for Disease Control and Prevention ART.
4. Brian Kearney, *High-Tech Conception: A Comprehensive Handbook for Consumers* (Bantam Books, 1998).
5. Susan Lewis Cooper and Ellen Sarasohn Glazer, *Choosing Assisted Reproduction; Social, Emotional & Ethical Considerations* (Indianapolis, IN: Perspective Press, 1998).
6. www.resolve.org—Resolve, the National Infertility Association.

CHAPTER 10

1. From the *Bhagavad Gita*.

Resources

FERTILITY-RELATED BOOKS

1. *Conquering Infertility* by Dr. Alice Domar
2. *The Infertility Cure* by Randine Lewis
3. *The Whole Person Fertility Program* by Niravi B. Payne, M.S.
4. *The Infertility Diet: Get Pregnant and Prevent Miscarriage* by Fern Reiss
5. *Wise Woman Herbal During the Child Bearing Years* by Susun Weed
6. *Taking Charge of Your Fertility* by Toni Weschler
7. *Infertility Sucks* Beverly Barna (humorous)
8. *Laughin' Fertility* by Lisa Safran (humorous)
9. *The Infertility Survival Guide* by Judith Daniluk
10. *Women's Bodies, Women's Wisdom* by Dr. Christiane Northrup
11. *Inconceivable: Winning the Fertility Game* by Julia Indichova
12. *Luna Yoga* by Adelheid Ohlig
13. *Stay Fertile Longer* by Mary Kittel
14. *Infertility Solutions* by Shana Albo
15. *Natural Solutions to Infertility* by Glenville (about diet)
16. *Making Babies* by Sami David
17. *The Infertility Survival Handbook* by Elizabeth Falker
18. *Is Your Body Baby-Friendly?* by Dr. Alan E. Beer about reproductive immunology
19. *Fully Fertile* by Beth Heller and Tami Quinn
20. *The Way of the Fertile Soul* by Dr. Randine Lewis
21. *The Mind-Body Fertility Connection* by James Schwarz
22. *Radical Acceptance: Embracing Your Life with the Heart of a Buddha* by Tara Brach
23. *Wild Feminine* by Tami Lynn Kent
24. *The Tao of Fertility* by Daoshing Ni and Dana Herko
25. *Fertility Wisdom* by Angela C. Wu

WEBSITES AND ORGANIZATIONS

1. www.yogaforfertility.net—Lynn Jensen's website
2. www.aspireyoga.com—Jill Petigara's website
3. www.mindandbodyfertility.com—Carol Knoph's website for Mind/Body Program for Fertility
4. www.resolve.org—RESOLVE, the National Infertility Association
5. www.goodtherapy.org—Association of Mental Health Professionals
6. www.asrm.org—American Society for Reproductive Medicine
7. www.npg-asrm.org—Nurses in Reproductive Medicine
8. www.arhp.org—Association of Reproductive Health Professionals
9. www.americanpregnancy.org—American Pregnancy Association
10. www.theafa.org—American Fertility Association
11. www.endometriosisassn.org—American Endometriosis Association
12. www.creatingafamily.org—a nonprofit providing education and resource for infertility and adoption
13. www.clearpassage.com—Fertility Abdominal Massage
14. www.pcosupport.org—Polycystic Ovarian Syndrome Association
15. www.nccaom.org—National Certification Commission for Acupuncture and Oriental Medicine
16. www.endocenter.org—Endometriosis Research Center
17. www.endozone.org—Where endometriosis patients find surgeons and solutions
18. www.Anjionline.com Fertility-specific meditations to download
19. www.natural-health-for-fertility.com—Positive affirmations for fertility
20. www.fertileheart.com—Julia Indichova's (author of *Inconceivable*) website
21. www.webmd.com/infertility-and-reproduction/default.htm—message boards run by MDs
22. www.invesp.com/blog-rank/Infertility—top 100 infertility blogs
23. http://100infertilityquestions.blogspot.com/—100 questions and answers about Infertility
24. www.early-pregnancy-tests.com/—inexpensive pregnancy tests, ovulation predictor kits, etc.
25. www.IVFconnections.com—resources for IVF and infertility
26. www.ivfmeds.com—London-based site for inexpensive IVF-cycle medications
27. www.babyhopes.com—site for inexpensive pregnancy tests in bulk
28. www.fertilityfriend.com—BBT tracking website
29. www.conceiveonline.com—website of *Conceive* magazine
30. www.fertilitylifelines.com—website of Gonal-f medication
31. www.repro-med.net/repro-med-site2/—Center for Reproductive Immunology and Genetics
32. www.arvigotherpy.com—The Arvigo Techniques of Maya Abdominal Massage Therapy
33. http://www.cdc.gov/art/—statistics for fertility clinic success rates

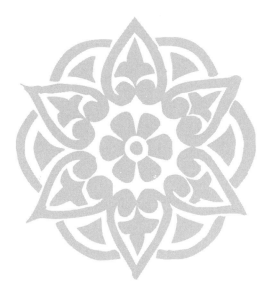

Index

abdominal massage, 20, 22, 225, 257–258
accept and respect, yoga principles, 23
acupuncture, 255, 256–257
aerobic exercise, 251
affirmations for fertility support, 238–239
alternate nostril breath, 230
apana, 11–12
ART, *See* assisted reproductive technology
Arvigo Techniques of Maya Abdominal
    Therapy™, 257
asanas, 225
assisted reproductive technology (ART), 206,
    255, 258–260
  clomid/IUI, 259
  collaborative reproduction/donor
    egg, 259–260
  IUI with injectable drugs, 259
  IVF, 259
avidya, 14
Ayurveda, 245

back poses, 104–110
basal body temperature (BBT), 21
belly breath, 38, 80, 126, 162, 181, 208, 229
benefits of yoga, 2–4, 16–17
bent knee twist, 43, 109–110, 134–135, 186,
    194, 218
blood flow, increased, 4–5
bloodstream, reducing stress hormones
    levels in, 6–7
BMI, *See* Body Mass Index
body
  apana and samana, 11–12
  energy balances in, 9–11
  life-force energy, 12
  listening to, 23–24
  mind and, 9
  regulation of, 3
Body Mass Index (BMI), optimal range of, 249
body-to-mind communication, during
    yoga, 23

bow pose, 101
breathing practices, 24, 228–230
bridge pose, 105, 185
    supported bridge pose, 207, 215

calming/centering breath, *See* centering/
    calming breath
calming effect, 139
    prayer pose, 48, 87
calm mind, 8–9
cat-cow, 45, 83, 136, 166, 196, 210
    circles, 46, 84, 137, 167, 197, 211
centering/calming breath, 38, 80, 126,
    162, 192
cervical mucus, 22
chakras, 5
chant, to support fertility, 241
"chicken wing" shoulder stretch, 35, 62, 123,
    148, 199, 213
child's pose, 31–32, 47, 50, 72, 86–87, 120,
    121, 138, 156, 169, 198
    restorative, 212
    variation of, 50, 103
Chinese medicine, 255, 256
    approach, 244
    fertility-supporting practices from, 257
Clear Passage Therapy™, 272
clomid/IUI, fertility treatments, 259
cobbler pose, 150, 201, 219
    with heart opener, 36, 63, 150, 182, 214
cobra, moving, 31, 51, 75, 100
collaborative reproduction/donor egg, fertility
    treatments, 258–259
coming up, 44, 61, 82, 110, 135, 195
conscious breathing practice for fertility
    support, 226–228
conscious mind, 9
corpse pose, 37, 39, 125, 153, 161, 189, 221
counseling and life coaching, 258
counted breath, 229

dharana, 225
dhyana, 225
digestive energy in the body, 11

downward facing dog, 31, 49, 50, 71, 85, 91,
    121, 140, 156, 168, 170

eagle arms, warrior 2 pose with, 74, 72
early pregnancy, legs up the couch pose,
    204–205
eight limbs of yoga, 225
emotional patterning, 14, 84, 137, 167, 197
emotional stresses, 5
endocrine systems, 50, 60, 68, 85, 99, 112,
    129, 141, 152, 168, 179, 215
    rebalancing, 14
    regulating, 5–6
endometriosis
    diagnosis of, 14
    treatments, 14–15
energy
    balances in body, 9–11
    feminine, 9
    increased, 4–5
    life-force, 11–12
essence, concept of, 253

feminine energy, 9
fertility abdominal massage, 20, 22, 255,
    257–258
fertility "altar," 239–240, 274
fertility issues, 256
    for hypnotherapy, 258
fertility nutrition
    ayurvedic approach, 245
    food sensitivities approach, 244–245
    lifestyle changes for, 243
    recommendations for, 245–247
    traditional Chinese medicine
        approach, 244
    Western dietician approach, 244
    "whole foods" approach, 245
fertility support
    affirmations for, 238–239
    conscious breathing practice for, 226–228
    meditations and visualizations for, 231
    practices from Chinese medicine, 257
    usefulness of yoga for, 11

"fight-or-flight" response, physiological changes associated with, 6
fish pose, 77, 106
folic acid, 246, 248–249, 269
follicle stimulating hormone (FSH), 259, 267, 271, 274, 275
forward bend over one leg, 159, 180–181
FSH, See follicle stimulating hormone

gentle seated twist, 202
goddess pose, 203, 209
groin stretch/lizard lunge, 73, 89

half-moon balance pose, 75, 96–97, 158, 174–175
hand and knee poses, 83–91, 136–142, 145–150, 166–170, 196–198, 210–214
happiness and the mind, 7
happy baby pose, 118, 132, 155, 165
hatha yoga poses, 2, 10
heart-to-uterus visualization, 237
hormonal system, imbalances in, 13–14, 16
hormone levels, impact on, 251
hypnotherapy, 255, 258

immune booster, wide standing forward bend with, 75, 98, 158, 178–179
infertility
    facts, 261
    unexplained factors of, 13–14
Intra Cytoplasmic Sperm Injection (ICSI), 259
intrauterine insemination (IUI)
    cycle, 268, 272
    with injectable drugs, 259
in vitro fertilization (IVF), 259, 273–274
    pose schedule for, 206–207
    process, 271
IUI, See intrauterine insemination
IVF, See in vitro fertilization

jing, 253

knee-down lunge, 33, 55, 72, 88, 121, 142
knee poses, hand and, 83–91, 136–142, 145–150, 166–170, 196–198, 210–214
knees to chest, 70, 81, 116, 127, 216

legs up the wall pose, 5, 20, 67–68, 79, 111–112, 124, 151–152, 161, 187–188, 206, 207, 226, 237
    early pregnancy, 204–205
less strenuous exercise program, 252
life coaching, counseling and, 258
life-force energy, 11–12
listening to the body, 23–24
L-methylfolate, 249
locust, 53–54, 102
lying on back, 39–44, 127, 128, 163–165

mala beads for meditation, 240
male fertility
    challenges, 16
    pose for, 223
mantras, 12, 20, 240
masculine energy, 9, 228
meditation, 7
    benefits of, 231
    elements of, 232
    mala beads for, 240
    mindful walking, 235
    passage, 236
    practices, 277
    seated, See seated meditation
methylenetetrahydrofolate reductase (MTHFR), 248–249, 276
    heterozygous for, 270
middle pain, See mittelschmerz
mind-body
    awareness, 19
    communication channel, 9
Mind-Body Fertility Connection, The (Schwarz), 238
mind/body program at fertility clinic, 267, 271
mind/body techniques, 17
mindful walking meditation, 235
miscarriage, 15

mittelschmerz, 22
"monkey mind," yoga, 8–9
monthly cycle, yoga routine, 19–20
mountain pose, 33, 56–58, 122, 143–144
moving bridge, 127, 128, 133, 154, 163
moving cobra, 31, 51, 75, 100
moving sphinx, 32, 52
MTHFR, See methylenetetrahydrofolate
    reductase

nadis, 4
negative thinking, reduction of, 8–9
niyamas, 225
normal-weight women, pregnancy in, 250
nutritional deficiencies, 247–249
nutrition, fertility, See fertility nutrition

outer hip stretch, 29, 41, 42, 118, 131, 217
ovaries, 5–6
ovulation, 21–22
    predictor kit, 22
oxytocin, 223

pancreas, 14
passage meditation, 236
pelvic areas, yoga for fertility increases, 4
pelvic floor contractions, 36, 64–65
    bridge pose prep with, 104
pelvic tension, 4
pelvic tilts, 29, 40, 77, 104, 118, 133, 160, 184
physiological changes, associated with
    "fight-or-flight" response, 6
    relaxation response, 7
pigeon pose, 73, 90–91, 157, 170
polycystic ovarian syndrome (PCOS), 14
practitioners, long-term yoga, 3
prana, 11–12
pranayama, 12, 222
    effects of, 228
    for fertility support, 226–228
prayer pose, 31–33, 47–48, 50, 54, 72, 76,
    86–87, 103, 120, 121, 138–139, 141, 156,
    169, 198
    variation of, 50, 103

pregnancy, 15
    mind/body techniques, 17
    in normal-weight women, 250
    problem, 256
    progression, 277
    test, 267
    yoga for, 204–205
pre-relaxation poses on the back, 184–186
principles of yoga, 23–25

Qi, acupuncture, 256

reclined cobbler pose, 42, 113, 203
regular yoga practice, 3
relaxation poses, 67–69, 111–113, 151–153,
    187–189
relaxation response, physiological changes
    associated with, 7
reproductive energy center, sacrum, 39
reproductive systems, 13, 14
    stimulation of, 5, 255
RESOLVE, national infertility
    organization, 258
restorative child's pose, 212
rest, yoga principles and, 24

sacrum circles, 28, 39, 117, 130, 154,
    164, 193
samadhi, 225
samana, 11–12
seated deep breathing, 228
seated meditation
    for calming, 234
    to clear the mind, 233
seated poses, 148–150, 180–181, 199–202
seated spinal twist, 36, 66
seated wide-leg straddle, 149, 183, 200
shoulder stand, 107–108
side angle pose, 93, 145, 171
sphinx, moving, 32, 52
squat pose, 146–147, 176–177
standing hip circles, 34, 57
standing poses, 56–61, 143–147, 181–179
stress hormones, reducing levels of, 6–7

stress reduction, 24, 206, 208
   massage and, 269
   exercise for, 252
subconscious messages, affect fertility, 238
subconscious mind, 9
suggestions, fertility, 260–263
supine poses, 51–55, 100–103
supported bridge pose, 207, 215

tension
   in pelvis, 4, 38, 42
   release from muscles, 41
   release by circling motion, 46
3-part abdominal breathing, 229
toxicity in body, 256
tree pose, 58, 144
triangle pose, 94–95, 172–173

ujayii (audible) breath, 228
uncomfortable feel in yoga practice, 24,
   95, 173, 239
unexplained infertility, factors of, 13–14
uterus
   endometriosis and, 14
   thickened lining of, 7, 21, 154

vigorous exercise, 250
   for stress reduction, 252

vision boards and fertility alerts, 239–240
visualizations
   for fertility support, 231
   heart-to-uterus, 237
vitamin B12, 248
vitamin D3, 247–248

warrior 2 pose with eagle arms, 92
weight and fertility, optimal range for, 249
wide standing forward bend, 59
   with immune booster, 98–99, 178–179
   with twist, 60

yamas, 225
yang energy, 10, 230
yin energy, 10, 230
yoga benefits, 2–4
yoga for fertility benefits, 3–4
yoga practice
   advantage of, 9
   basic principles of, 25
   deep breathing and, 126, 162
   for early pregnancy, 204
   recommendations for, 222
   regular, 3, 7, 15, 17
   uncomfortable feel in, 24, 95, 173, 239
yoga principles, 23–25
yoga routines, 20–22, 191
yogurt, 246

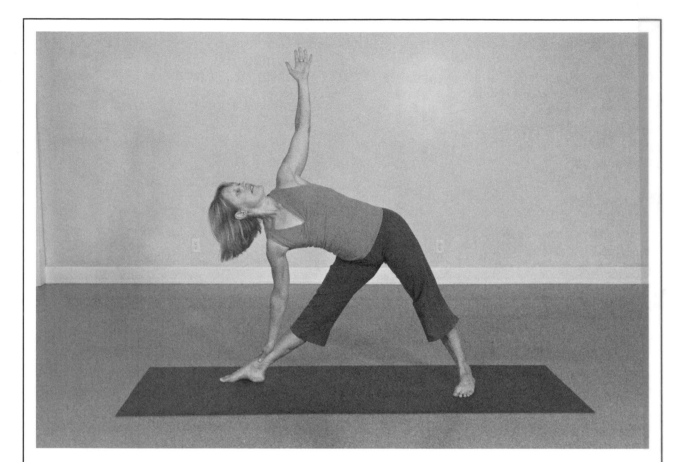

Yoga and Fertility DVD

Join Jill and Lynn as they lead you through easy-to-follow *Yoga and Fertility* routines designed around your monthly cycle. Choose from basic or intermediate level routines, specifically created to support ovulation, conception and implantation while promoting the body's relaxation response. The routines include breathing practices, fertility-enhancing yoga poses, and guided relaxation.

To order or download the DVD, or for a quick preview, visit our websites:
www.yogaandfertilitydvd.com

Practicing *Yoga and Fertility* is an important step on your fertility journey!

Namaste,
Jill Petigara, E-RYT, and Lynn Jensen, E-RYT, RPYT